ENERGY FOR LIFE

How to Overcome Chronic Fatigue

OTHER VITAL HEALTH PUBLISHING/ ENHANCEMENT BOOKS TITLES

Nutrition in a Nutshell: Build Health and Slow Down the Aging Process, Bonnie Minsky, L.C.N., M.A., 192 pages, 1-890612-17-0, $14.95.

The Cancer Handbook: What's Really Working, edited by Lynne McTaggart, 192 pages, 1-890612-18-9, $12.95.

Wheatgrass: Superfood for a New Millennium, Li Smith, 164 pages, 1-890612-10-3, $10.95.

Stevia Rebaudiana: Nature's Sweet Secret (3rd ed.), David Richard, includes stevia growing information, 80 pages, 1-890612-15-4, $7.95.

Stevia Sweet Recipes: Sugar-Free — Naturally! (2nd ed.), Jeffrey Goettemoeller, 196 pages, 1-890612-13-8, $13.95.

Taste Life! The Organic Choice, Ed. by David Richard and Dorie Byers, R.N., 208 pages, 1-890612-08-1, $12.95.

Lecithin and Health, Frank Orthoefer, Ph.D., 80 pages, 1-890612-03-0, $8.95.

Natural Body Basics: Making Your Own Cosmetics, Dorie Byers, R.N., 88 pages, 0-9652353-0-0, $9.95.

Anoint Yourself With Oil for Radiant Health, David Richard, 56 pages, 1-890612-01-4, $7.95.

My Whole Food ABC's, David Richard and Susan Cavaciuti, 28 color pages, children's, 1-890612-07-3, $8.95.

The Veneration of Life: Through the Disease to the Soul, John Diamond, M.D., 80 pages, 1-890995-14-2, $9.95.

The Way of the Pulse: Drumming With Spirit, John Diamond, M.D., 116 pages, 1-890995-02-9, $13.95.

The Healing Power of Blake: A Distillation, edited by John Diamond, M.D., 180 pages, 1-890995-03-7, $14.95.

The Healer: Heart and Hearth, John Diamond, M.D., 112 pages, 1-890995-22-3, $13.95.

Life Enhancement Through Music, John Diamond, M.D., approx.172 pages, 1-890995-01-0, $14.95.

ENERGY FOR LIFE

How to Overcome Chronic Fatigue

Dr. George L. Redmon, Ph.D. N.D.

VITAL HEALTH PUBLISHING
Health ~ Nutrition

It is not the intent of the author to diagnose or prescribe. Nor is it the purpose of this book to replace the services of your physician. This material is intended for educational purposes only. It is advisable to seek a doctor for any condition that may require his or her services.

Energy For Life: How to Overcome Chronic Fatigue
George L. Redmond, Ph.D., N.D.
Copyright 2000 © George L. Redmond, Ph.D., N.D.

Printed in the United States of America by United Graphics, Inc., Mattoon, IL on recycled paper using soy-based ink.

Published by:
Vital Health Publishing
P.O. Box 544
Bloomingdale, IL 60108
www.vitalhealth.net
vitalhealth@compuserve.com
(630) 876-0426

ISBN: 1-890612-14-6

ACKNOWLEDGEMENTS

I am greatly indebtly to Ms. Suzan Windley, Mr. Eric Dettrey and his secretarial support staff, especially Lorri Fioravanti, for the exceptional editorial and copy work done on this manuscript.

I also wish to express my deep and lasting appreciation to my editor, Mr. David Richard of Vital Health Publishing, for his consideration in providing the platform for this presentation's review and study. Additionally, this researcher would like to thank Mr. Richard for his input, enthusiasm and guidance in the preparation of this manuscript.

I am sincerely grateful to the past and present researchers who have laid the groundwork and foundation which has spawned a new era of acceptance for natural and alternative healthcare. I also am sincerely grateful to the following individuals who have supplied the emotional fuel, and in some cases their expertise and knowledge, without which this project could not have been completed.

Dr. Lloyd Clayton
President
Clayton College of Natural Health
Birmingham, AL

Dean Eugene Jones
Continuing Education Department
Burlington County College
Pemberton, NJ

Dr. Barry Pensky, E.D.
New York City University
Department of Education
New York, NY

Dr. Willard E. Downham, Jr., E.D.
Director of Adult School
Washington Township Public School
Sewell, NJ

Ms. Andrea Foster, Director
The Holistic
Resource and Referral
Network of Houston, TX

Dr. Marcia B. Steinhauer, Ph.D.
Department of Health And Human Services
Walden University
Minneapolis, MN

DEDICATION

This book is dedicated to my wife Brenda, whose undying love and devotion has been and continues to be an inspiration and strong motivating force in my everyday existence.

— Dr. George L. Redmon, Ph.D., N.D.
September, 1999

Philosophically, the ideas at the foundation of Western Medicine are called deterministic and materialistic, and they're based on nineteenth century Newtonian physics, which say that reality is composed of pieces of matter that bounce into each other like balls on a billiard table. But the physics of Einstein, known as quantum physics, paints a very different picture of reality. You know its central formula: $E=MC^2$. What this formula means is that all matter is nothing but a dense version of energy or light. And this energy or light is an eternal substance that never dies, but that constantly changes into many forms.

— From *New Choices in Natural Healing*

Table of Contents

PROLOGUE

"The discrepancy between the prevalence of chronic fatigue in our society and the abundant energy in the natural world creates a troubling paradox. It is puzzling to say the least. With so much energy throughout nature, how can anyone possibly feel fatigued? Why is fatigue a daily experience for millions of people? Why, for many of them, is it the dominant experience of their lives? The most perplexing question, however, in this paradoxical paradigm (model) is why do the overwhelming majority of people who suffer with chronic fatigue have no clear physical cause for their problem?"

Dr. Deepak Chopra, M.D.
World Authority on Aryuvedic Medicine
Boundless Energy

"Physicians would rather deal with an identifiable disease than an illness. If your doctor responds to your symptoms of fatigue by acting as though you are an impossible complainer, because they can't be proved physiologically, you might remind the doctor that until the connection between the pancreas and sugar metabolism was discovered, doctors considered diabetes to be a psychological disorder."

Miryam Ehrlieh Williamson
Fibro-Myalgia: A Comprehensive Approach,
What You Can Do About Chronic Pain and Fatigue

"Too often when no physiological conditions are detected, the patient may be told that they are perfectly healthy and that there is no reason to be concerned. Although the person may feel better to find out that there is no apparent physical condition causing their fatigue, they are left to deal with the situation on their own. They *suffer* in silence."

Dr. Holly Atkinson, M.D.
Former Medical Reporter for CBS News
Women and Fatigue

"This is an unfortunate error doctors sometimes make assuming that fatigue, not obviously physical in origin, may be psychological. There is a false dichotomy (something between mutually exclusive groups) in that belief, which pervades all areas of medicine that whatever is not on the medical maps, is in the province of psychology. There is, however, another possibility that the fatigue a patient is suffering is in the 'Terra Incognita of undiscovered knowledge about the body'."

We need to explore that Terra Incognita!

Dr. Ronald Hoffman, M.D.
Medical Expert on Human Energetics
Tired All the Time

PREFACE

In Search of Energy

My search for energy began some 20 years ago after I battled and won my fight against Hodgkin's Disease. Hodgkin's Disease is a form of cancer that attacks the lymphatic system. The lymphatic system is a vital part of the immune system that directly affects the body's ability to produce a strong immune response. Untreated, this disease can render the body helpless to ward off and fight foreign invaders. Without treatment, death eventually occurs.

Some years ago, this malady meant certain disaster, but today, with early detection, this disorder can be contained and rendered harmless. The standard medical treatment is through radiation and chemotherapy. Both of these protocols tend to have a devastating affect on individual energy levels and, paradoxically, can depress the immune response. Other complications of this form of treatment include (although not in all cases): severe weight loss, loss of appetite, loss of taste, constant regurgitation, dehydration and extreme fatigue.

The Cure, Almost Worse than the Disease

After several weeks of radiation treatments, doctors insisted that my system had been eradicated of this disease and within a few months, I would regain my strength, the weight I had lost, my hair and my natural skin tone. Sure enough, those regenerations did occur, but with two glaring problems: drastically reduced energy levels and a diminished capacity to ward off colds and other infections. I was instructed to get plenty of rest and to consume a variety of different foods. Also, doctors suggested that when I felt very lethargic, I should come in for what was referred to as "booster" shots.

This routine, however, proved to be less than satisfactory and I began my quest to understand the world of "Human Bioenergetics". In addition to searching for a better long term solution to fading energy levels and a faltering immune response, I discovered some astonishing things. For example, when I used supplemental enzymes in my dietary regimen, my energy level significantly increased. I also found that by—

- incorporating an antioxidant formula into my diet regimen, my energy level increased.
- starting to use a multi-vitamin and mineral formula, my energy and immune response improved.
- following a cycle of natural detoxification measures, I felt a lot more energetic.
- replacing or incorporating more fresh raw fruits and vegetables on a daily basis, I felt more energetic.

What was so exciting about these developments was the fact that not only did my energy and immune response show short-term improvements, short-term became mid-term and mid-term became long-term. Today I am vibrantly energized, but more importantly, I am still learning. I have spent the last twenty years learning how to continuously improve my immune response and cultivate the internal bioenergetic system nature has provided me with.

The Energy Roller Coaster

According to Karen Collins, M.S., R.D., of the American Institute for Cancer Research, a typical day for people on an "energy roller coaster" starts with some energy, but by mid-morning they have bottomed out. If you are one of the millions struggling to start your internal engine in the morning, desperate to keep it running after lunch, and only too willing to let it sputter or die in the evening, you are not alone. In fact, according to recent reports by the Centers for Disease Control, this phenomenon of diminishing energy levels has escalated in the last few years and needs to be studied in greater detail.

Dr. Deepak Chopra, M.D., a world authority on the "Mind-Body" connection, states that "despite the fact that fatigue is widespread in modern life, it really is a unique phenomenon when seen in the context of "nature". Dr. Chopra maintains that the elements of nature all around us are dynamic and represent a tremendous constant flow of energy and activity. Dr. Chopra goes on to say "physicists insist that the universe is nothing other than one dynamic pulsating field of overwhelming energy." Researchers insist that energy is constantly around us, being endlessly converted from one form to another, although we cannot see, touch, feel or smell it.

A Monumental Question

If the universe is nothing more than one high-powered force of interminable energy, *independent of life,* with life (each of us) however completely dependent upon it and its dynamic force, **How Do We Capture, Harness and Unlock Its Potential?**

Flora Davis, the author of *Living Alive,* maintains that "human energy" is an astonishingly complex and powerful spectacle. A force that is very much underestimated, misunderstood and often under-utilized. She maintains that many people feel that energy (or vitality) is just a matter of what you eat and how often you exercise, with sundry psychological factors thrown in.

A Question of Energy

Just what is energy? What color is it? How is it formed and structured? Where does it come from? Why does it come and go, sometimes in abundance and at other times, seemingly non-existent?

Is it hot or cold? Can it be measured? Can I alter or manage its potential? Should I expect it to diminish as I age? Can it be stored? Am I born with a lifetime supply of it?

In my search for answers to the above questions and others, the one word that has stuck out in my mind over this twenty-year search is "potential". When viewing energy in the context alluded to by Dr. Chopra, one can see that nature is *an inexhaustible conglomeration of power and dynamic cycles of orderly, structured and timely bursts of energy*. Knowing how to unlock the biological potential of the unlimited supply of energy that nature has made available is the key to sustaining and maintaining peak energy levels.

A Question of Potential

The word potential is defined as something capable of coming into actuality or realization. Potential is also described as a latent (concealed or dormant) excellence or ability that may not be developed. Fatigue is defined as a feeling of lethargy, tiredness or physical and mental weariness, while energy is defined as the capacity of matter to perform physical work or an organism's ability to participate in or perform vigorous activity.

As energized matter, we therefore possess the ability to perform physical work and participate in vigorous activity. However, we are subject to feelings of fatigue and the suppression of overall development of our full energy potential. In effect, we are subject to the elements of change as described below by Dr. Andrew Weil, M.D., one of the world's foremost authorities on alternative medicine.

The Elements of Change

Change is a factor that affects our daily lives. Our bodies are subject to dramatic internal and external cycles of change such as aging, illness, seasonal changes in the weather or everyday stress. These incidences of stress and change can interfere with the balance or equilibrium that our internal systems wish to maintain, thus affecting our energy level and feeling of well being. Dr. Weil states that "during these times of internal change or disturbed equilibrium, healing comes from inside and not outside. It is simply the body's natural attempt to restore balance when balance is lost."

The key question then becomes, how do we unlock and harness the energy potential that naturally surrounds us, which helps support and maintain our delicate internal equilibrium?

Unlocking the Potential

We are but a mere miniaturization in the evolving fabric of nature. We exist as cubicles, part of nature's biological scheme, in which we are used to perpetuate, store, and transfer energy and the vital life forces which preserve its existence.

Since energy can't be created or destroyed in matter, but only transferred, we are subject to the laws of this natural transference, so possessing the ability to continuously unlock the potential of the non-quantitative force known as "energy".

In other words, we are transfer agents or chemical stations, with a potentially unlimited energy supply. We are, however, bound by the natural forces and dynamic actions of the environment. The way in which we respond, interact and abide by this dynamic interaction in part will determine how well and how efficiently this innate energy potential manifests itself.

It is nature that provides, but we who determine the eventual outcome. As expressed by Dr. Rob Krakovitz, M.D., a board member of the Orthomolecular Society and an expert who specializes in "metabolic nutrition":

Energy is your birthright. Unless there are special genetic or congenital problems (which are extremely rare), you are born with the potential to have all the energy you will ever need.

Dr. George L. Redmon, Ph.D., N.D.
Advisory Board Member
Clayton College of Natural Health
Sicklerville, New Jersey, 1999

INTRODUCTION

Everyone from time to time feels fatigued, but are you finding it harder and harder to bounce back? Have you recently been to your doctor due to a lack of energy or even an overall feeling of discontentment? Are you tired when you get up in the morning, tired at mid-day and just generally exhausted at the end of a normal day? To make matters worse, have you had x-rays and lab tests done which revealed that there is nothing physically wrong with you? If you have answered 'yes' to any of the above questions or fit the above profile, you may definitely be a victim of the "Human Energy Crisis".

According to the editors of the *Doctor's Book of Home Remedies*, Rodale Press, Emmaus, Pa., 1990, "fatigue may be just a signal that you need to manage your life better, or that a cold or flu is coming on." It can also be a sign of serious illness. "Anything that is chronic — diabetes, lung disease or anemia — will cause fatigue", says Dr. Rick Ricer, M.D., an assistant professor of clinical family medicine at Ohio State University College of Medicine in Columbus, Ohio. Dr. Ricer also maintains that fatigue can be a symptom of many other illnesses including hepatitis, mononucleosis, thyroid disease and cancer.

It is advisable if you have persistent chronic fatigue that you discuss this with your health professional. Persistent fatigue and loss of energy is not normal.

Energy, An Elusive Entity

Based on current data, researchers have concluded that there is a real energy crisis on the horizon. This impending crisis is not connected with the price of crude oil or the rising cost of gasoline or home heating oil. This energy emergency is "human" in nature and has become a real issue as we head into the twenty-first century. In fact, reports out of the Center for Disease Control (CDC) in Atlanta have described a type of recurring fatigue known as the "Chronic Fatigue Syndrome."

Researchers describe this malady as an unrelenting, continuous episode of exhaustion. Some symptoms of this disorder are:

- Increased thirst
- Poor sleep patterns
- Recurrent infections
- Exhaustion after minimal efforts
- Depressed immunity
- Bowel disorders
- Aches and pain
- Forgetfulness
- Anxiety and depression
- Hormonal imbalances

As reported in the *Journal of the American Medical Association*, three to six million Americans suffer from this disease. According to Dr. Ronald Hoffman, M.D., Medical Director of the Hoffman Center for Holistic Medicine in New York City, there are no specific tests to "prove" you have this syndrome. Because of this, it is diagnosed by symptoms that severely restrict normal activity and are not due to other diseases.

Two other common symptoms according to the Center for Disease Control are:

- Fatigue for at least six months, usually of rapid onset; fatigue that lasts twenty-four hours or longer after exercising.
- Sore throat and painful lymph nodes in the neck.

However, there is a large percentage of Americans who suffer from a general feeling of fatigue, tiredness, weakness and listlessness, who do not fit or have the unrelenting symptoms expressed by the CDC. A recent public health report revealed that only one in 13,535 people who suffer from symptoms of fatigue meet the CDC guidelines. Health officials, however, contend that Americans today make over 500 million office visits to doctors every year to complain about the negative effects of generalized fatigue.

When You Are Tired and Don't Know Why

Although fatigue is something regarded as a symptom rather than a treatable condition, it can have as devastating an effect on a person's quality of life as the most concrete surgical disorder according to Dr. Denton A. Cooley, M.D., Surgeon-In-Chief at the Texas Heart Institute. Dr. Cooley goes on to say that since fatigue is hardly life-threatening, and since it is a condition that even healthy persons frequently experience, it is tempting to regard tiredness as simply being part of the human condition.

Dr. Richard N. Podell, M.D., (Department of Family Medicine, University of Medicine and Dentistry of New Jersey) states that this is the position taken by many physicians. Dr. Podell maintains that instead of taking the patient's condition seriously, many doctors see it as a "complaint", and become very impatient with chasing the elusive symptoms of fatigue.

An even more insidious fact is that the broad prescription offered by many doctors — get plenty of rest, eat a balanced diet and exercise — will have little or no effect in changing the continuous cycle of exhaustion, weakness and fatigue for millions who struggle with its debilitating effects every day.

Fatigue is Real

Because this cycle is such a normal part of daily life, it is something we don't think about, according to Dr. Holly Atkinson, M.D., a former medical reporter for "CBS Morning News" and author of *Women and Fatigue*. We may only realize we feel too much of it at certain times and at other times we may not even be fully aware that we are fatigued. Getting to know your own fatigue and the fatigue of those close to you can help your life run more smoothly. To properly address your fatigue level, you need to start paying close attention to all of the sensations (mental and physical) that make up your present condition.

The Meaning of Energy

For most of us, having enough energy means feeling good enough to accomplish the tasks of our everyday lives to be able to do the things we need without feeling excessively tired afterwards. If, however, you are one of the growing number of Americans who struggle with the negative effects of fatigue for no apparent reason, you are not alone.

Your Energy Potential

Health experts contend that that each of us has an inherent energy potential pool that we were born with. This pool represents the amount of energy on which we might have to draw during the day. We start out with a certain level of energy that comes from our natural reserves. Here, natural reserves refer to the amount of energy contained within a living body. To a certain extent, scientists claim that this natural reserve is dictated by heredity. For example, some people seem to need a few hours of sleep, while others need more; some are always bursting with energy, while others tend to drag through life. I believe, however, that in today's high tech chemical society, natural reserves of energy are drastically altered causing metabolic imperfections thus limiting our ability to realize our full energy potential.

Energy is the essence of life. Without it you cannot function effectively or achieve your goals. Your ability to manage this vital natural resource has a direct effect on your physical, mental and emotional well being. For many individuals in search of energy, life has become a nightmare. Throughout my years of experience as a Holistic Health Counselor, in talking to thousands of consumers, I have found this problem to be almost universal. I have found it to affect individuals from all walks of life and from all age groups, even young teenagers as well as adults of all nationalities. These people, I believe, are within a limited existence, never realizing their full energy potential. However, most of us are born with the ability to utilize nature's unlimited energy supply to lead whatever kind of life we choose. In fact, most of the time we draw on only a minute fraction of our true energy converting capabilities.

To make the most of your life, you really need to make the most of all the energy you were born with.

As previously stated, the variables that can interrupt the dynamics of the human energy cycle are seemingly infinite. Nevertheless, to properly manage your innate energy potential, how well you are able to control many of these variables will determine how energetic you will be. However, as stated by Dr. Michael Colgan of the Colgan Nutritional Institute in San Diego, CA.:

Reaching your goals while combating the possible pitfalls of maintaining a healthful and energetic existence is no longer your trainer's or physician's battle, it is yours.

The Purpose of this Book

I believe that fatigue is not a normal condition. As stated by Dr. Rob Krakovitz, M.D., "under normal circumstances you are born with the potential to have all the energy you need." Furthermore, while many health professionals maintain that you are born with a certain energy potential, Dr. Robert Willix, who developed the first open-heart surgery program in South Dakota, states that, "not only are you born with an innate energy potential, you control it." To help you to assess the overall ramifications of this topic, I have divided this book into two sections. The first section, which includes Chapters one through three, looks at the "Nature of Energy". This section reviews:

- Just exactly what energy is.
- The biological need for energy.
- Where it originates.
- The role of the cell in energy production.
- How it is captured and stored by natural means.
- How energy is transferred and transformed throughout nature and in living systems.
- How energy is made available for human use.
- How and where energy is oxidized (burned) to supply fuel to the body.
- The major internal energy molecule known as "ATP".
- The different classifications that are given to energy.

- The concept of "thermo-dynamics" and its relationship to the overall pool of available energy throughout the universe.

Section two, "Managing the Potential of Energy", which contains Chapters four through eight, shows you how to control and manipulate your full potential of energy. Some topics covered in section two are designed to show you:

- How to manipulate your food intake to insure that energy levels are maintained throughout the day.
- Many health rejuvenating secrets from around the world.
- How to establish your own individual fatigue profile.
- How to determine your real biological age, to assess your personal youth quotient.
- Some of the most widely used natural energizers on the market today.
- How to set up and establish a long range supplement plan based on your own individual needs.
- How to track and set your own food-mood clock to perform at peak levels throughout the day.
- New frontiers concerning nutrient absorption rate.
- How to increase your immune response two-fold as well as how to slow down your internal "biological clock".
- Why intestinal cleansing is important to maintain peak energy output.
- How to stimulate and develop good digestion, a key factor in the metabolic process, and maintenance of superior energy levels.

Energy For Life: How to Overcome Chronic Fatigue is concerned with moving you from a one dimensional model to a holistic approach in overcoming fatigue.

Dr. Stephen Schechter (*Fighting Radiation and Chemical Pollutants with Foods, Herbs and Vitamins*, 1994) remarked that to produce a continuous cycle of energy, it is important to take a "comprehensive approach". *Energy For Life: How to Overcome*

Chronic Fatigue will show you how to boost your energy levels by using a comprehensive approach that is fun and exciting. You will be able to set up short-term, interchangeable goals that are designed to provide energy when conditions create new demands, as well as for daily living. A brief synopsis of each chapter follows:

CHAPTER 1 — Investigates the need for constant energy and its role in sustaining bodily functions and life. The goal of this chapter is to define just what energy is, its origin, its chemical make-up, its mode of transference and its transformation. The concept of potential energy, as well as the difference between chemical and physical energy, is also explored. The overall purpose of this chapter is to review how the cycles of energy originate in nature.

CHAPTER 2 — Reviews how nature has provided each of us with an inborn metabolic mechanism. When we follow applicable guidelines as nature intended, internal metabolic cycles will function at peak levels. The purpose of this chapter is to explain how and where metabolic energy is produced internally. The aim of this section of the text is to assess the actions of the internal metabolic pathway known as the "Krebs Cycle".

CHAPTER 3 — Examines the concept of fuel and how power is produced from that fuel. The purpose of this chapter is to review the special organelles located in the cells known as the "mighty mitochondria". It is in the mitochondria where glucose, fatty acids, and amino acids are transformed into the energy rich molecule known as "ATP" (Adenosine Triphosphate).

CHAPTER 4 — Focuses on energizing food concentrates. The goal of this chapter is to examine which foodstuffs are considered to be energizing. Daily caloric intake, basal metabolism (how the body uses calories for energy), food combination, the food pyramid guide and the glycemic index of foods are discussed. Also, a basic overview of governmental nutritional standards as well as recent research out of M.I.T. (Massachusetts Institute of Technology) and other leading institutions concerning the food/mood/mind response and its direct relationship to overall energy levels is revealed. The goal here is to examine how manipulating certain brain neurotransmitters (via food) can increase energy levels.

CHAPTER 5 — Deals with the use of various natural supplemental programs and products designed to augment a balanced food program. This chapter looks at the use of vitamins, mineral, herbs and their relationship to the human energy cycle. This section also examines the role of amino acids in relationship to energy and reviews "The Central Fatigue Hypothesis", which suggests that central fatigue is a sub-set of fatigue that is associated with specific alterations in "CNS" (Central Nervous System) function. Additionally, this segment of the book also reviews the overall importance of detoxification programs as well as physical exercise's role in the preservation and maintenance of one's energy potential.

CHAPTER 6 — Looks at the issue of premature aging, a strong immune response, and its relationship to the human energy cycle. This chapter also summarizes the free radical theory of aging and the role of antioxidants, considered by many health officials to be the most important medical discovery in the last fifty years. Lastly, Chapter 6 shows the reader how to determine their need for antioxidants and helps them to assess their real biological age.

CHAPTER 7 — Teaches the reader how to determine their own individual fatigue profile. The purpose of this chapter is to help the reader identify many possible "energy drainers" and "energy boosters" in their lives, which will enable them to pinpoint areas of concern. Furthermore, this chapter reviews the mechanisms of stress and theories of Hans Selye, known as the "Father of Stress Response". The intent here is to show the reader how stress can wreak havoc on energy levels.

CHAPTER 8 — Puts it all together. The purpose of this chapter is to demonstrate how a "Management Model" is constructed. By formulating organized scenarios of goals and activities, "action plans" with attainable energy producing objectives can be established. This section also informs the reader of several different energy-enhancing programs as outlined by some of the most respected authorities on the subject of human energy enhancement.

The overall objective is to show the reader how to build one's very own individualized energy plan, focusing on long term energy-enhancing objectives via short term interchangeable "action plans" and goals.

Section One

The Nature
of Energy

"Matter and energy, the two go dancing off together to form our cosmos — matter the substance, energy the mover of the substance. But this dualism is a very sophisticated idea and the concept of energy itself is a relative newcomer in the edifice of knowledge. Unseen and untouched, almost certainly energy can only be imagined in the mind of a man or woman. How it came to be conceived in all its complexity and how it came to be put to work in our everyday lives constitutes one of the greatest detective stories in the history of science."

Mitchell Wilson
Rene Dubos
Henry Margenall
C.P. Snow
Time-Life Science Library
Energy

Chapter One

DEFINING ENERGY: ITS POTENTIAL AND BIOLOGICAL NEED

"Energy is constantly being changed from kinetic (energy in motion) to potential (stored or inactive) and back again. The biological world is no exception. Living organisms operate by changing potential energy found in foodstuffs into kinetic energy of muscle contraction and the manufacture of needed structural parts. Energy is independent of life. Life, however, is completely dependent upon energy".

Baker and Allen
Matter, Energy, and Life

According to Dr. Albert P. Mathews, Ph.D., a former Carnegie Professor of Biochemistry, living things have five major properties. These properties are movement, growth, reproduction, respiration (the taking in of oxygen and giving off carbon dioxide), and irritability. Irritability here refers to the ability to adapt to changes within the environment.

How living things can do these things has only become the subject of innumerable studies in recent times. Dr. Mathews makes note of the fact that since living things are apparently lifeless things plus "something else", it was assumed that there was in living things a spirit, an energy, an entelechy or demon. It was not until the end of the 18th century that this explanation was doubted.

The Study of Human Bioenergetics

When you review the remarks by Dr. Mathews, they imply that the study of "human bioenergetics" is relatively new, new in the sense that it has only been in the last eight or nine decades that some clear-cut answers have begun to emerge in solving the mysteries of how plants, animals and human beings capture and utilize this invisible entelechy known as energy.

The Energy Burden

For most of us, energy means feeling energetic enough to complete our daily tasks without undue weakness. While we may have enough energy to do the above, researchers contend, however, that most of us never realize, reach or utilize our full energy potential. As stated by the biochemical researchers, Baker and Allen, quoted in the opening caption of this chapter:

"Energy is absolutely necessary to fuel life's processes, although it is not dependent on those processes to exist."

Just what is energy?

- How does energy enter the system?
- What does it do for us?
- Can it be stored for future use?
- Why do scientists classify energy under different headings or by different types?
- What does potential energy mean?
- Does the body create or produce energy as it is needed and, if so, where does this occur?
- Is it produced twenty-four hours a day or only at certain intervals throughout the day or night?
- How is energy controlled and used?

Human Bioenergetics

Scientists have, for some time, been investigating how the body maintains itself and all of the forces necessary to fuel and sustain its everyday needs. A general term used to describe the many ways our body extracts and uses energy is referred to as "energy metabolism" or "bioenergetics". The science of bioenergetics as we know it today was initiated with the studies of Lavoisier (1743 – 1794) who discovered the principles of "in vivo" (live tissue) and "in vitro" (test tube) oxidation and combustion.

Another early researcher named Von Liebig, whose studies have been credited with having just as much significance as those of Lavoisier, showed that carbohydrates, fats and protein were oxidized (combined with oxygen) in the body, not combined with hydrogen and carbon as thought by Lavoisier. Lavoisier misinterpreted how protein was used as an energy source and believed that its catabolism (breaking down) was caused only by muscular work. It was not until nearly fifty years later, about 1900, that Von Liebig showed that protein metabolism (break-down) was not exclusively related to muscular work. During this same time period, Rubner in 1901 conclusively demonstrated the validity of the laws of conservation of energy in intact (whole) animals.

Human Energy, its Origin, Cycle and Transformation

Scientists now know that we do not have the capability to create our own energy. Energy is transformed from one kind to another and is transferred for use everywhere on earth. This is known as the law of thermodynamics and coincides with the law of conservation of energy in living things.

Since living things are constantly in motion, growing, changing shape and size, reproducing and adapting, there is always a need for energy. Although it was once believed that energy was regulated by some unknown force or spirit, this myth has been dispelled. Researchers now know that human energy has a primary origin, and that origin is the distant, yellow, glowing star we call the sun.

Let the Sun Shine In

Scientists have discovered that energy will only flow in one direction, from forms that have abundant energy to forms having less usable stores of it. This latter description refers to us. Energy as we know and feel it flows to us from an outside source. We do not create it. That outside source, namely the sun, fuels all the processes of life.

Within the framework of the natural flow of energy, all living matter (including ourselves) serve as miniature holding tanks or devices that permit nature to recycle energy to preserve it and do its work. We serve as machines that transform chemical energy and other kinds of potential energy into kinetic energy (energy in motion). Kinetic energy can appear as heat, light (as when lightning bugs light) or electrical energy. Some examples of the electrical energy generated in your body are the impulses that keep your heart beating or the transmission of signals between your nervous system and your brain.

It would appear from our discussion thus far that energy originates from the rays of the sun and that it is transferred from somewhere else. But from where, and what is the sun's role in this process? Also, other key questions that arise are:

1. How is energy from the sun captured, stored, unlocked and transferred for biological use?
2. Is energy actually created, destroyed and recreated or is it simply recycled?
3. If we cannot create energy, then what is it that gives us energy? Are our internal organs being energized or is it something else?
4. What are the different forms of energy?

The Seat of Transformation

To fully understand the importance of the sun's role in determining your present energy levels, let's see if we can form a model of the transformation of its combustion. The process goes something like this:

Step 1. As the sun shines, its radiant energy is captured and stored in plant life. It is within the green pigment or color in plants, called chlorophyll, that this radiant energy is transformed into life-sustaining chemicals. This is controlled by very small substances (molecules) called chloroplasts, which contain the pigment chlorophyll.

Figure 1.1 that follows shows exactly what is going on inside those green leaves during the photosynthesis process.

The Plant as a Factory

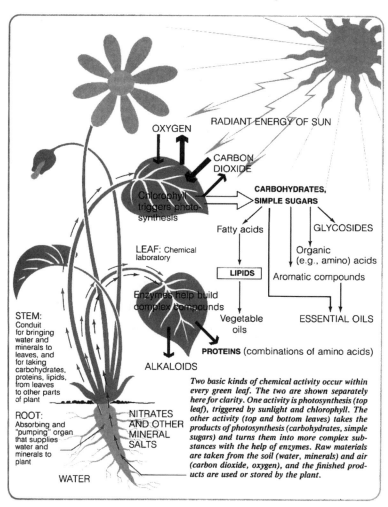

RADIANT ENERGY OF SUN

OXYGEN

CARBON DIOXIDE

Chlorophyll triggers photosynthesis

CARBOHYDRATES, SIMPLE SUGARS

Fatty acids

GLYCOSIDES

LEAF: Chemical laboratory

Organic (e.g., amino) acids

LIPIDS

Aromatic compounds

Enzymes help build complex compounds

Vegetable oils

ESSENTIAL OILS

STEM: Conduit for bringing water and minerals to leaves, and for taking carbohydrates, proteins, lipids, from leaves to other parts of plant

PROTEINS (combinations of amino acids)

ALKALOIDS

ROOT: Absorbing and "pumping" organ that supplies water and minerals to plant

NITRATES AND OTHER MINERAL SALTS

WATER

Two basic kinds of chemical activity occur within every green leaf. The two are shown separately here for clarity. One activity is photosynthesis (top leaf), triggered by sunlight and chlorophyll. The other activity (top and bottom leaves) takes the products of photosynthesis (carbohydrates, simple sugars) and turns them into more complex substances with the help of enzymes. Raw materials are taken from the soil (water, minerals) and air (carbon dioxide, oxygen), and the finished products are used or stored by the plant.

Figure 1.1 Source:
The Readers Digest Association, Magic and Medicine of Plants, Pleasantville, NY, 1989, p. 43

Let The Sun Shine In

Figure 1.2 below further illustrates this sequence of events. This entire process is known as photosynthesis. When the sun is shining and radiant energy is being transformed, these reactions are called light reactions. Light reactions enable or start the cycle in which light or radiant energy is converted to different forms for use by all living organisms.

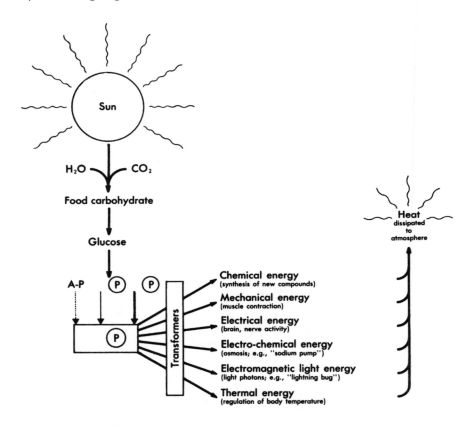

Figure 1.2 Source:
Sue Rodwell Williams, Essentials of Nutrition and Diet Therapy, C.V. Mosby, Co., 1978; p. 26, 27

The Approach of Sundown

Step 2. We now know that the rays of the sun are vital and serve as the catalyst or driving force in energy production and its transformation.

How does this process of energy production continue to fuel life's processes when the sun goes down? In essence,

HOW IS RADIANT ENERGY FROM THE SUN TRANSFORMED INTO CHEMICAL ENERGY TO ENERGIZE THE FOODS WE CONSUME THAT FUEL METABOLIC PROCESSES THAT PROVIDE ENERGY TO HUMAN TISSUE IN THE ABSENCE OF SUNLIGHT?

The Dark Reactions and ATP

As described in Step 1, deep within the recesses of the green pigment found in a chloroplast, nature converts this radiant or light energy from the sun into electrical energy. It is this electrical energy that keeps all of our bodily processes, from our heart- beat to our muscular contractions, in working order. This, in turn, results in the generation of chemical energy, which is the energy your cells need to do their work. In this process, an energy-rich molecule named "adenosine triphosphate" (sometimes called the "energy current of life" or "ATP") supplies the energy or fuel necessary to allow these so called "dark reactions" to occur.

Energy Never Stops Working

Researchers have found that the need for energy is constant and ongoing. The reactions previously described occur every day, 365 days a year, every hour and every minute, somewhere in nature. In fact, in the presence of sunlight, also known as the sparking phase, electrical energy is converted into chemical energy in a hundred millionth of a second in the plant kingdom.

At this point, the body is able to oxidize food molecules (when combined with oxygen) into energy-rich nutrients that have been created by radiant energy from the sun. This process, however, needs some help. This help comes from enzymes. Enzymes are proteins that act as catalysts. That is, they can accelerate the action of a reaction without being used up by that same reaction.

In essence, enzymes keep the energy process moving. Without them, these reactions would not occur, at least not at a rate sufficient to fuel the biological requirement for energy in living organisms. We will discuss in more detail the use of supplemental enzymes and other metabolic enhancers in chapter five, "Natural Energizers". At this point, it is important to be aware of how the process of photosynthesis is related to the formation of "ATP", your energy molecule.

The Green Grocer

This process that starts at the light of day is a reciprocal one between the sun — plants — and ourselves. From this perspective, one can see that energy does not exist in a vacuum.

Dr. Henry Bieler (*Food is Your Best Medicine*) uses the following equation to illustrate one aspect of the energy cycle:

Energy + NCO2 + NH2O – NO2 + CNH2NON ....(1)
CNH2ON – NH2O + NCO2 + Energy ....(2)

The scientific formula aside, it is only important to remember reaction (2) in the above graphic is the opposite of reaction (1). The first of the two reactions is performed only by the chlorophyll-containing plant cells, while reaction (2) is performed by all cells, whether of the plant itself, the animal which eats the plant (herbivore), or the animal which eats the animal which eats the plant (carnivore). In each case, there are certain natural reactions that will occur, producing energy within the organism when certain conditions exist and certain key elements are present.

A Natural Biological Cycle

It is *foods* that the plant and animal kingdom use to provide us with the potential energy that radiates from the sun. This natural occurrence, in scientific terms, is intertwined with the laws of thermodynamics and the conservation of energy in living things, which I mentioned earlier. In reality, when you view energy from this standpoint, it is everywhere and remains constant. A general overview of these standard laws of nature and their relationship to "human bioenergetics" is cited in the subsequent paragraphs.

The Law of Thermodynamics

There are actually two laws of thermodynamics and the first one deals with the quantity of energy available. It is expressed in this way.

The total amount of energy in the universe remains constant. More energy cannot be created and existing energy cannot be destroyed. It can only undergo conversion from one form to another.

In other words, whenever and wherever the energy conversion takes place, the total energy of the system and its surroundings (the environment), after the conversion, is equal to the total energy before the conversion took place. This is what is meant by a reciprocal process. Energy was captured, converted and used by one system (namely you), but during the process, its by-products (waste such as carbon dioxide expelled from the lungs) is returned to the environment to be recycled. This lays the groundwork for the process to repeat itself.

The Energy Pool Always Remains the Same

The biological researchers, Starr and Taggart, authors of *Biology – The Unity and Diversity of Life,* 1987, Wadsworth Publishing tell us that there is a definite amount of energy in the universe. It is distributed among various forms, such as the chemical energy stored in molecular bonds and the radiant energy from the sun. According to the above authors, these and other forms of energy are interconvertible. For example, plants absorb sunlight energy and convert it to the chemical energy of sugar. You eat plants and the chemical energy stored in sugar can be converted to mechanical energy that powers your movements. Some energy escapes into the surroundings as heat during these conversions. Because of ongoing conversions in your cells, your body steadily gives off the same amount of heat as a hundred watt light bulb. However, none of the energy vanishes. More precisely, the total energy content of a body and its surroundings remain constant.

The Second Law of Thermodynamics

The second law of thermodynamics centers on the notion of the direction in which energy flows, involving energy exchanges. Because of this, researchers refer to it as "time's arrow". The second law states that:

In all energy exchanges and conversions, if no energy leaves or enters the system, the potential energy of the final state will always be less than the potential energy of the initial state.

In other words, energy flowing from a source provides the source and activates the potential energy of something else. For example, heat will flow from a hot object to a cold one, but not the reverse. In human terms, we can utilize the radiant energy from the sun only by eating plants that have captured and stored the energy. Or we can utilize the potential energy of food and cells by eating animals, which have fed on the plants that again, have captured and stored the energy of the sun's rays.

Figure 1.3 which follows, takes a look at this concept of recycling matter and energy.

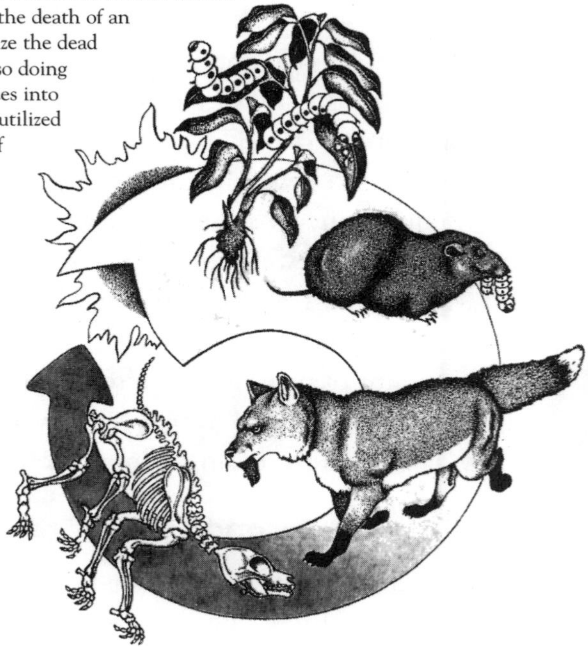

Recycling matter and energy through a small portion of the living world. Plants convert light energy into chemical energy in the nutrients they synthesize. Herbivores such as caterpillars utilize plant material for a source of nutrients and energy and are themselves used by carnivores such as the shrew. Other carnivores such as the fox feed on lower level carnivores. Upon the death of an organism decomposing organisms utilize the dead body for nutrients and energy and in so doing break down complex organic substances into simple inorganic compounds that are utilized again by plants during the synthesis of new nutrients.

Figure 1.3 Source:
Jack A.Ward, Howard R. Hetzel, *Biology Today and Tomorrow*, 2nd Ed., West Publishing Co., 1984, p. 6

Energy and Death

From the above graphic, we can see that even in death, the decomposing elements are returned to nature for recycling. This again shows us that energy remains constant and that its original pool can't be destroyed. The molecules released at death provide raw materials that fuel newborns, future generations and nature's perpetual existence.

The key is to give the body what it needs and let it decide how to transform and use the energy. We will cover this in more detail in chapter four "Food Is Your Best Medicine". However, to fully realize your full energy potential according to how these energy transformations (which occur endlessly in nature) affect your metabolic pathway, it may be wise to learn as much as you can about how it works.

Conclusions

When we go back and review the opening remarks made by the biochemical researchers, Baker and Allen, we can now see why life (including ourselves) is totally dependent upon energy. The cells of our body need fuel to do their work (chemical work) in order to supply us with the needed energy to do our physical work. Cells use and need energy to:

- Build and repair tissue
- Remove cellular waste that can poison the body and cause disease
- Protect the body against bacteria and viral invasion
- Assist cells in their effort to communicate problems to one another to help maintain your internal balance known as homeostasis

When the body is functioning at peak capacity at the cellular level, it is meeting practically all of your biological need for energy.

Robert Crayhon, cited as one of the top ten nutritionists in America, maintains that energy is crucial for health. He states that nearly every great medical tradition in the world is built upon the axiom of nurturing the natural energy/vitality within. This is something completely different from "stimulant" energy. Mr. Crayhon cites the fact that when we are tired, we can rest, but if an individual cell runs out of energy, it dies. If this process occurs at an accelerated rate, not only will your energy level decline, but your overall health and well-being will be severely compromised.

In the next chapter "Nature's Energy Blueprint" we will take a look at where in the body cellular energy transformations take place.

NATURE'S ENERGY BLUEPRINT

"Studies show that in all cells the molecules of electron-transport chains are placed next to one another in definite patterns to form assembly lines that yield "ATP". This suggests that the controlled flow of charged particles in animal and plant cells, in living as well as man-made electronic systems, apparently requires a fixed arrangement of components and a specifically designed circuitry. One of the most significant advances in the rapidly advancing life sciences is the discovery that nature has built its own carefully constructed electronic devices into all organisms."

John Pfeiffer
Former Science Editor of *Newsweek*
Former Science Director, CBS

Change is a factor or variable that affects our daily lives. Our bodies are subject to dramatic internal and external cycles of change such as aging, illness, seasonal changes in the weather or everyday stress. These periods of change can interfere with the balance or equilibrium that our internal systems wish to maintain, affecting our energy levels and feeling of well being. The living forces inside the cell utilize a tightly organized system of parts to sustain it. Dr. Andrew Weil, M.D., believes we should be conscious of the dynamics of these internal changes. Dr. Weil states that "due to all the forces we are subjected to, it is nothing short of miraculous that the body is able to sustain itself ". Additionally, maintaining the dynamic interplay of this fixed arrangement of components and specific internal circuitry that Mr. Pfeiffer describes is crucial to sustaining energy for both chemical and physical work. The following are some important questions regarding our internal energy circuitry.

- What are cell organelles?
- What is the goal of cellular oxidation?
- How is energy organized, gathered and transferred?
- What is ATP and why is its production or yield important?
- What are living forces inside the cell?
- What role do they play in energy production?

Chapter two will focus on answering these and other pertinent questions.

The Electrical System

When an electrician needs clarification regarding the operation and construction of a piece of electronic equipment, the most widely used diagram to retrace its intended course of action is the "blueprint" "or" "schematic". A schematic is used for analyzing, explaining and servicing circuits and proposed maintenance of an operating system. In many cases, symbols are used in electronic diagrams because experience has shown that they are the quickest and most efficient way to convey the needed information. Simple symbols are a form of electronic shorthand. With them a circuit can be sketched in a short time; and because the symbols are standard, other persons can easily interpret them.

Figure 2.1 shows the schematic of a typical amplifier used in a portable phonograph. The schematic shows all the electrical components and how they are connected to make up the circuit. The value (size) or type of each component is given, along with the colors of transformer leads, the connections to each and other identifying marks. Additionally, a chart showing electrical measurements obtained at the various points and the conditions under which they were taken can also be seen.

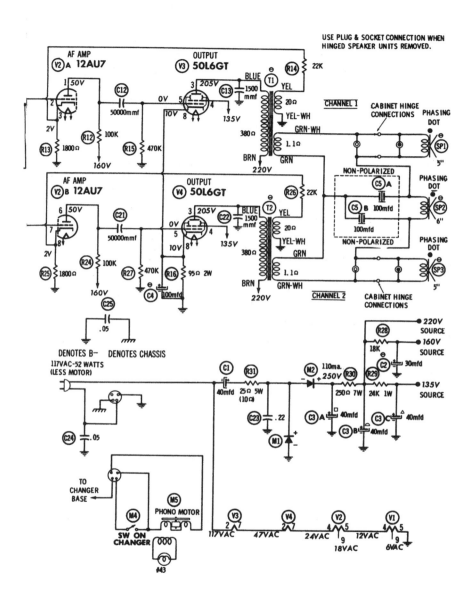

Figure 2.1 Source: Donald E. Hennington, *Schematic Diagrams,* Howard W. Sams and Co., Inc., Indianapolis, In - 1970, P. 7

I have chosen this schematic representation to give you an idea of the dynamic interplay of our own inborn energy processing system. For just as this blueprint or schematic of the phonograph represents a working plan to control energy transformations, a similar design can be developed that represents our own internal metabolic energy system. In both types of systems (man-made and innate human systems) as stated by John Pfeiffer, electron-transport chains form precise patterns, which control the flow of charged particles. This example illustrates that when certain compounds, components or elements undergo change, the energy produced in this transference must have some orderly pattern to initiate, engage and ultimately produce or provide an efficient energy source.

When Worlds Collide

It is at this level where biology and electronics intersect. The existence of electrical energy producing processes in "human bioenergetics" carries with it certain characteristics, as is represented in the diagram of the man-made schematic of the phonograph. It is very important to note here that within human bioenergetics, although nature has supplied us with a unique inborn energy blueprint, the blueprint however doesn't produce the energy. This concept coincides with the working of the blueprint of the phonograph. The blueprint allows the phonograph to be built but it doesn't play music. Conversely, the genetic code in our cells (DNA and RNA) allows the cell to be built. However, the genetic code doesn't directly process energy, the cell does.

The Living Forces Inside The Cell

Although cells vary widely in their shape, all of them have four basic components and can be compared to an industrial plant. The cell has:
- A central control point (the round ball of the nucleus)
- Power plants (the mitochondria)
- Internal communication stations (the cytoplasm containing various organelles vital to the cells operations)
- Construction and manufacturing elements (the jelly-like mass known as the protoplasm)

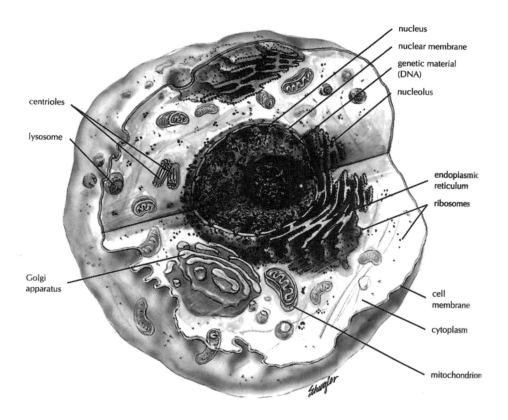

Figure 2.2 Source: Hemmler, Cohen, and Wood, *The Human Body in Health and Disease*, Lippincott, Plilladelphia, PA - 1996, P. 28

Cellular Organelles

Just as you have various organs within your system, such as the liver, kidneys, heart and spleen, each one of those trillion cells in your body also have their own organs or "organelles". Each of these organelles has specific responsibilities that ensure the health and energy capability of the cell is maintained, as do your internal organs. The following table gives a birds-eye view of the functions of the various organelles found in your cells. (See Table 2. 1)

CELL STRUCTURE AND ACTION

Structure	Function
Nucleus	Controls cellular activities and reproduction of Eke cells
Nucleoplasm	Constitutes the environmental medium of the components within the nucleus
Chromatin	Substance Carrier of genes, i.e., units of heredity, in dispersed form in resting cell
Chromosomes	Condensed chromatin substance, carrier of genes during cell division
Nucleoli	Produce cytoplasmic ribosomes (see below); provide plans or templates for synthesis of ribosomal RNA
Nuclear membrane	Controls interchange of materials between nucleus and cytoplasm
Cytoplasm, cytoplasmic structures	Metabolism, transport, and reproduction
Cytoplasm	Forms the inner structure of the cell
Mitochondria	"Powerhouse" releasing energy to carry out work of the cell
Ribosomes	Protein synthesis
Endoplasmic reticulum (granular)	Transfer and delivery system of ribosomes
Golgi complex	Assembly site for various secretions
Lysosomes	Packaging and strong intracellular digestive enzymes
Centrioles	Participate in cell division and are apparently associated with development of cilia, hair cells in the ear, and light-receptive cells in the eye

Table 2.1 Source:
King and Showers, Human Anatomy and Physiology W.B. Saunders, Philadelphia, Pa - 1969, P. 31

As you can see, the cell can be compared to a busy metropolis whose needs to generate power are constant. All in all, good cellular health is important to our own individual energy production. But the work cells must perform also requires energy. Mr. Pfeiffer also notes that the existence of electrical energy within the cell carries certain implications. He goes on to say "sustained electric currents in the cell cannot be produced by some hocus-pocus maneuvers". Thus the need for specialized units in its energy-producing processes is as important as that found in man-made electronic circuitry.

The Human Bioenergetic Maze

This organized sequence of electrical activity, which is vital to the formation of compounds and molecules that produces energy to sustain life's vital processes, is depicted by the following blueprint or schematic. (See Figure 2.3)

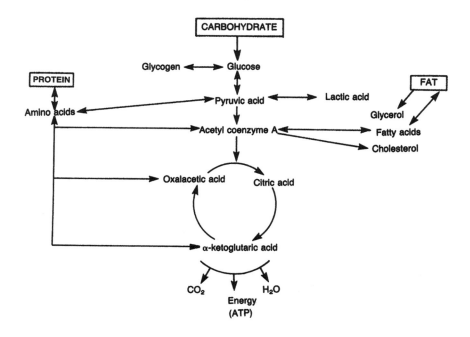

Figure 2.3 Source: Garrison and Somer, *The Nutrition Desk Reference*, Keats Publishing, New Cannan, CT - 1995, P. 20

This natural conversion of power, the transfer and creation of major energy molecules, begins in the mouth (when you consume food) and ends with a series of dynamic movements through a "metabolic maze". Scientists refer to this as metabolism or "energy metabolism". As depicted in Figure 2.3, macronutrients (carbohydrates, fats and proteins) are broken down into their component parts. Carbohydrates are converted to glucose (sugar) and fat to glycerol (a triglyceride) and fatty acids. Proteins are broken down into amino acids. After these macronutrients are synthesized and enter the bloodstream, they are carried to the liver and then to various tissues and cells by the blood stream. Once in the cells, these nutrients are chemically transformed by the metabolic process of oxidative (mixing with oxygen) reduction, energy release, synthesis (combining separate parts or elements to form a whole) and finally storage. Nutrients consumed in excess of immediate energy or building needs are stored as fat for later use. Contrary to popular belief, protein (amino acids) not used for repair of bodily structures and tissues is also stored as fat.

There Is Unity In Nature

Besides the macronutrients, the integrity of this metabolic maze known as the "citric" or "tricarboxylic acid cycle (TCA)" is also dependent on vitamins, minerals, enzymes and various hormones. These nutritional components play a major role in energy metabolism. They assist in an array of organized reactions that release the potential energy from food. As such, these other components are considered essential to the chemical liberation of energy, thus also having a role in maintaining physical energy.

This cycle of events is also known as the "Krebs Cycle", named after the German-born biologist who first suggested the existence of this dynamic metabolic pathway in 1937.

The Goal of Cellular Oxidation

Scientists now know that the major goal of the body in this orderly, systematized routing is to produce "energy molecules". The major molecule is "ATP", scientifically known as "adenosine triphosphate". In fact, you could say that your body lives and breathes to produce this energy molecule.

The two well-known biochemists, Pearson and Shaw, state that, "ATP is the substance which stores the energy that is created when the body burns carbohydrates and fats within our inner energy blueprint". When energy is needed by the body in, for example, a muscular contraction, ATP is broken down to release the stored energy. ATP is the universal energy molecule for your body in the same way that electricity is the universal energy source for a computer.

However, the breakdown and conversion of ATP to supply energy is a continuous process. There is no on or off switch as with your computer and its electrical supply. This precious stuff (ATP) is essentially your raw power source, and when there is a need for energy to make the heart beat, to expand the chest in breathing, or to blink an eyelid, ATP breaks down into simpler substances, releasing energy as it does. As long as you live, there will be this call for "energy" and "ATP". Even in the deepest sleep, there is continual activity as cellular furnaces burn to keep your body warm and your heart cells pulsing, pumping the rivers of your blood.

The Life Span of a Cell

Every second, fifty million of your body cells die. In this second, some fifty million infant cells are also born to take the place of the dying cells. All this movement and activity in the cell require constant energy and our biological quest for survival turns into a series of attempts to acquire and harness the energy necessary for existence. This search for energy, this constant movement, the tidal wave of material passing through our body's metabolic pathway and being manipulated, converted, turned upside down, torn apart and pieced together again, forms the dynamics of life.

Conclusions

The biological molecule "ATP" is always available to release its energy rapidly and explosively whenever needed by the cell. It also is important to remember the word "structure". Your internal energy mechanism is always working hard to maintain its proper structure and its systematic routine that astonishingly occurs every minute.

Nature's Master Plan

As we have learned, nature has already installed an elaborate mechanism to insure that your energy needs are met. Conversely, nature has provided you with a controlled cycle of events that are designed to provide you with an unlimited energy potential. However, in order to unlock this potential energy, the dominant chemical energy of our foods must have a means to be converted to live substances. Substances need to be ingested which are capable of yielding the necessary energy for cellular work (chemical energy) that will in turn provide enough energy for you to sustain yourself and your ability to do physical work.

A Few Unanswered Questions
- Where does energy metabolism take place?
- What molecules are formed from ATP?
- What elements play a key role in this conversion process?

Investigations into this phenomenon have revealed that there are tiny structures or organelles within the cell where our internal fuel is burned and electricity is literally produced.

In the next chapter, we will take a look at these tiny power-houses where nature uses (oxidizes) food to yield the rich energy molecule "ATP". We will also take a closer look at our metabolic blueprint to find out why scientists contend that within the confines of this natural schematic there is always "energy to burn".

Chapter Three

ENERGY
TO BURN

"Every day the average man and woman uses up enough energy to bring at least thirty-five quarts of ice water to a boil."

Isaac Asimov
Former Professor of Biochemistry
Boston University School of Medicine
Chemicals of Life

These remarks by Isaac Asimov, the famed science writer, imply that the human body uses and has a tremendous capacity to store energy. They also imply that the human body has the ability to convert energy into heat, enough to raise a static cold temperature to a fiery boiling one. However, as cited by Dr. Lawrence E. Lamb, M.D., former professor of Medicine at Baylor University and Chief of Medical Sciences at the School of Aerospace Medicine, it is an outdated misconception that food is burned with oxygen in the cells. With this in mind, when we go back and take a look at the source of energy in our solar system, the sun, the word "transfer" comes to mind.

It is in this context that energy is utilized. The body actually transfers energy back and forth in its chemical compounds. Researchers maintain that the body's continuous attempts to make and transfer energy molecules is the foremost or "second most" function of every cell. However, according to Dr. Lamb, it takes an enormous amount of energy to move chemicals throughout the cells (energy metabolism) and maintain life processes as well as supply you with the energy to do your work. When you view energy in this context, several key questions come to mind:

- How does the body make energy?
- Is there a chemical name for energy?
- What is oxidation?
- How is heat produced?
- What is energy metabolism?
- What is meant by life processes?
- What are enzymes and hormones and what role do they play in energy production and utilization?

As stated earlier by Dr. Flora Davis, author of *Living Alive*, "human energy is an astonishingly complex and powerful spectacle". This thought, coupled with professor Asimov's remarks, make it clear that, despite popular belief, the greatest concentration of energy is not in the Middle East, it lies somewhere within you!

Bioenergetics in Action

Energy as it relates to the human body, can be separated into two broad categories: chemical and physical. You use energy to walk, exercise, or carry out your daily activities. This is "physical" energy. A cell also uses energy to make things happen, as when it constructs large molecules from smaller, simpler ones. This is chemical energy. It is through this dynamic cycle that our bodies live and breathe to produce life's internal energy molecule known as "ATP" (adenosine triphosphate), which is covered in detail within this chapter.

Hatfield and Zucker, the authors of *Improving Your Energy Levels Nutritionally*, also remind us that the ATP contained in the cells is the body's energizer and that it is broken down through a variety of enzymatic processes. During this process, sparks of energy are released that stimulate hundreds of microscopic filaments and cross-strands within each cell, triggering contractions. According to Hatfield, this chemical act is repeated endlessly and your body eats, drinks, and breathes to perform it.

To fully understand the concept of energy, let's take a closer look at these two concepts. The biological researchers Starr and Taggart note that one of the most difficult connections to make is the link between yourself — a living intelligent being— and such obscure terms as metabolic pathways, cells, hydrogen, carbon, oxygen and nitrogen. These elements and concepts are however the "stuff" or "material" you and your energy system are made of. They are the reason why you are alive.

This energy, needed by your cells, is referred to as "chemical energy". When the cells produce this chemical energy to perform their duties, the body uses it to perform your physical work. This refers to your ability to walk, run, exercise, have sex, and carry out your other normal activities. Chemical energy is directly produced from the food you eat.

According to Dr. Lamb, also author of *Metabolics: Putting Your Food Energy to Work*, the body is a remarkable processing plant. There is a processing unit to break down chemicals and another to assemble new compounds, such as protein for enzymes and hormones. Dr. Lamb goes on to say that, "just as you can use wood, coal, gas or electricity to produce heat, the body can use fats, carbohydrates, or proteins to produce energy. The body has a remarkable ability to simplify the process which converts all the different foods we eat to a few simple compounds that eventually are processed in the same way."

In fact, researchers know that this organized sequence of events requires an input of chemical energy. Chemical energy is the energy of food and fuels, or more precisely, the energy contained in chemical molecules. Thus, the chemical energy of food molecules is liberated (released) by catabolic (breaking down) oxidative reactions. It is this input (when you eat) of chemical energy (food) that enables the cell to make biological molecules. These reductional (when food is broken down) and oxidative (when food mixes with oxygen) events are the key principles of biochemical energy production or human bioenergetics. How well you are able to meet the constant demand for energy to sustain the processes of life has a critical impact on your overall energy levels and the maintenance of your health.

Chemistry 101- The Elements of Life

There are many elements that occur widely within nature. Present knowledge or scientific inquiry has isolated over 100 of them. Elements are the mineral salts found in nature and in our bodies. To produce energy, the body must have a way of using these elements in an efficient manner.

Naturally occurring elements are commonly found in all living things. They cannot be broken down into substances with different properties. Different elements can combine in fixed and unchanging proportions to form what scientists call "compounds". For example, the compound water has a fixed proportion of two elements: 11.9% hydrogen to 88.1% oxygen by mass. Table 3.1 lists the elements most common in living things. Note the chemical symbols for each element and their abundance in the human body. (See Table 3.1)

Atomic Number and Mass Number of Elements Commonly Found in Living Things				
Element	Symbol	Atomic Number	Most Common Mass Number	Abundance in Human Body* (% Weight)
hydrogen	H	1	1	10.0
carbon	C	6	12	18.2
nitrogen	N	7	14	3.0
oxygen	O	8	16	65.0
sodium	Na	11	23	0.15
magnesium	Mg	12	24	0.05
phosphorus	P	15	37	1.1
sulfur	S	16	35	0.25
chlorine	Cl	17	35	0.15
potassium	K	19	39	0.35
calcium	Ca	20	40	2.0
iron	Fe	26	56	0.004
iodine	I	53	127	0.0004

Source: Starr, C., Taggart, R., *Biology: The Unity and Diversity of Life*; Wadsworth Publishing, Belmont, CA, 1987, p.36

This data shows that the three most concentrated elements in your body are oxygen, hydrogen and carbon, which make up 93% of it. Much of the oxygen and hydrogen is linked together in the body in the form of water. However, researchers now know that these two elements are also bonded together in considerable amounts to carbon which is the most important structural component in the body.

When united with oxygen, hydrogen will generate energy. In human systems, this and the carbon combinations are how energy is produced. A reaction that initiates a reduction change in the molecular structure of the agent or compound in question is known as "oxidation".

Molecules: The Essence of Life

All living things grow and maintain themselves in the form of molecules. A molecule is a unit of two or more atoms (the smallest unit of an element) of the same or different elements bonded together. Current research concerning this natural metabolism suggests that a high level blueprint of interconnecting circuitry can be found at the molecular level. Oxidation occurs when molecules are catabolised (broken down) into carbon dioxide and water. Without oxygen, this process cannot happen. During this oxidative process, energy is released from food which is the energy that allows our cells to do their work. This energy also supplies us with our vitality, vim and vigor. It allows our bodies to do their physical work.

Putting The Oxidation Process in Motion

Before the oxidation process can occur to produce energy, two things must be available. First, there must be fuel present, and second oxygen must be at hand. Since we have no way of storing oxygen, nature has some built-in mechanisms that allow us to store appreciable amounts of carbohydrates and fats. Oxygen is readily available in these substances for our use.

When you cook at home, you simply turn up the power to increase the energy or heat of your range. There is no flame, however, burning in your energy system. Through a series of organized events, the body slowly breaks down the energy molecules of fats and carbohydrates. This ensures that energy isn't released all at once, instead yielding an even flow of heat and energy.

The Biological Transformation of Energy

A general term used to describe the many ways your body extracts and uses energy from the foods you eat is called "energy metabolism". As discussed in Chapter One, the breakdown of fats, carbohydrates and proteins into their usable forms happens via metabolic pathways. These breakdowns are done in a series of stages; each one dependent on completion of the previous stage. This cycle of events is referred to as life processes.

To fully understand the importance of this concept, visualize the following, which could be described as "accessing your energy system".

Let's say that you can only get into your house by walking up and opening the gate that surrounds it. If for some reason your key will not open the gate, you can't get to the front door to enter the house. In the above scenario, what is missing is the right key and/or combination of keys. Enzymes are the biological 'keys' that jump start your energy metabolic cycle. They ensure that each cycle occurs and is completed before the next stage can begin. Like most things in nature, enzymes do not work alone, and often need the help of vitamins and minerals. Hence, the need to incorporate supplemental enzymes and vitamins and minerals into your diet. They help to keep your energy system firing on all cylinders, much the same way 'spark plugs' do in a car. They are in essence the switches that control your internal energy system. They provide the spark that ignites your energy system into action.

The Worksite

As we discussed in Chapter Two, the body is constantly manufacturing the energy molecule ATP through an orderly sequence of events known as the Kreb's cycle. Let's look more closely at this process.

ATP is the powerful body fuel that the cell uses for all of its functions. In essence, ATP serves as an energy reservoir and goes through endless cycles of catabolism and anabolism . In fact, the energy that is locked up in an ATP molecule is not stored for any length of substantial time. Typically, the energy in an ATP molecule is consumed and unleashed within sixty seconds of its formation. Even if you were bed-ridden for twenty-four hours, your cells would turn over about four kilograms (a unit of mass and weight equal to 4000 grams) of ATP molecules just for normal maintenance.

Because of the endless creation and re-creation of ATP, it is also referred to as "the internal flame of life", or "the energy current of the cell", *for the body cannot work at all except by using ATP.*

ATP Creates Muscular Contractions

Figure 3.5 below shows that adenosine tri-phosphate (ATP) is made up of adenine (a nitrogen-containing compound), ribose (a five carbon sugar); and three linked phosphate groups (a triphosphate). One or more of these phosphate groups, as discussed earlier can be transferred to another molecule (such as glucose [sugar]). In this case, ATP then becomes ADP (adenosine diphosphate – two phosphate). This molecule (in this case sugar) to which the phosphate group becomes attached is said to have undergone "phosphorylation". (See figure 3.5)

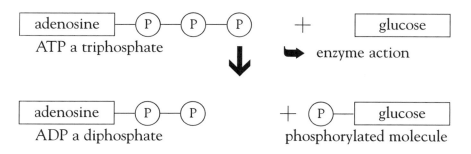

Source: Starr, C., Taggart, R., *Biology: The Unity and Diversity of Life;* Wadsworth Publishing, Belmont, CA, 1987, p.105

Researchers have confirmed that during this transfer and binding to phosphorous, the energy stored in these molecules increases, preparing them for specific biochemical reactions.

Starr and Taggart, authors of *Biology: The Unity and Diversity of Life*, state that many different molecules can be phosphorylated by ATP and liken this process to the currency of a gold coin, rather than say, a dollar bill or peso, since gold is accepted as a currency in any country in the world. They go on to say that almost all metabolic pathways rely, directly or indirectly, on ATP — truly nature's biological gateway to interminable energy.

So as you can see, the largest concentration of energy lies within you, not in the Middle East. In fact, deep within the recesses of the human cell (some 60 trillion in the body) there are powerful ATP generators or powerhouses known as the "mitochondria".

Your Internal Powerplant

The mitochondria can be described as super-minute, sausage shaped power stations that process energy, produce electricity and leave "wet ash" (water and carbon dioxide) behind.

Scientists contend that mitochondrias are so elaborately designed that they can be said to be cells within cells. According to John Pfeiffer, author of *The Cell*, and a former science editor for *Newsweek*, the interiors of the mitochondria look something like cut-away models of ocean liners with many chambers and compartments that have dividing walls. Although miniature in stature, these internal power plants provide the cell with the energy it needs for growth, reproduction and other functions.

Please see p. (23) in Chapter Two to get an idea where mitochondria are located within cells and how they look.

Understanding the Importance of Mitochondrial Function

To understand the importance of the mitochondria, think about the enormous amount of power generated to keep an entire city lit at night. The job of the mitochondria can be compared to that of your local electric company, except the raw material used to produce energy (electricity) is the food absorbed by the cell. It is in the mitochondria (the cellular powerhouses) where food is broken down to form "ATP", freeing energy stored in these macronutrients by transforming them into a usable form.

As stated by biological researchers King and Showers, the mitochondria provides the chemical energy for active transport, synthesis, and all enderogonic (energy requiring) and exergonic (energy yielding) chemical reactions. The mitochondria also provide the platform for the conversion of factors into energy for mobility, contraction of muscle, and for transmission of nerve impulses. In fact, if a continuous supply of ATP were not produced in the mitochondria, initial levels would be used up. This would prohibit the formation of new ATP and chemical energy, causing diminished or altering physical energy. If left unchecked, all cell functions would stop, causing the cell (and eventually the body) to die.

To reiterate a fact previously mentioned, the body cannot work or function at all except by using the "ATP" molecule. The energy stored in the ATP molecule actually runs many of the body's metabolic functions and pathways. However, this mitochondria activity occurs 24 hours a day, 365 days a year, to insure your bioenergetic pathway is not compromised.

Unleashing ATP's Dominant Force

Scientists have discovered that when the body catabolizes carbohydrates, proteins and fats, the energy derived from this process is used to form several high-energy compounds. The metabolic reactions concerned with the conversion of these broken-down food molecules into larger molecules is known as "anabolism". Anabolism is involved with the body's repair and rebuilding phase of tissue structures and the formation of and transformation of biochemical energy, according to Drs. Montgomery, Conway and Spector of the Department of Biochemistry at the University of Iowa College of Medicine.

The high-energy compounds formed during the process described above are known as "phosphates". Phosphates are readily found in soil fertilizers. In the human body they are found in the bones. In fact, one sixth of the weight of the bones is phosphorous. The rest of the phosphorous (a mineral element) is found in some of the most important protein molecules in the body. The phosphate that contains the least amount of energy is called "adenosine monophosphate" (AMP). In this union there is one compound of adenosine bound to one unit of phosphate.

When a unit of adenosine is combined with two phosphate units it is called "adenosine diphosphate" (ADP). This additional bond contains much more potential energy.

Finally, during this conversion or interchange of chemical energy, a combination of one adenosine unit and three phosphate units is created forming "ATP" (adenosine triphosphate).

Conclusions

We are, in one sense, chemical factories that can transform potential energy into usable forms of energy. In this process thousands of reactions are simultaneously occurring. Is this why energy levels are at their Himalayan peak sometimes and at others as low as Death Valley? In practical terms, no. There are many factors that can interfere with the proper transference of energy, which we will cover in subsequent chapters.

Basically, our cells need fuel to do their work. In fact, as cited by Dr. Robert Crayhon, considered to be one of the most knowledgeable nutritionists in America, when we are tired, we can rest. But if an individual cell runs out of energy, it dies. If cellular attrition occurs at an accelerated rate, body processes will slow down and so will your vitality.

The key is to give your body the raw materials it needs and let it decide how best to use them to create energy. This is the focus of our next chapter: "Proper Nutrition: Your Best Energy Source". Please read on and find out why researchers claim that you actually control your own energy potential!

Section Two

Managing the Potential

Against the back drop of a nutrition science seemingly created for the benefit of the food industry, there arose a counter-movement of health professionals who were learning that nutrients had therapeutic effects. I became a part of that movement, and I am pleased to have helped thousands of doctors join the groundswell of those who recognize vita-nutrients to be a tool of healing. Nutrition is now poised to replace pharmaceuticals as the primary treatment choice in medicine.

Dr. Robert C. Atkins M.D.
Founder and Director
The Atkins Center

Chapter Four

PROPER NUTRITION, YOUR BEST ENERGY SOURCE

"Food is far more important than just something you eat for pleasure or to appease your hunger. Rather, it is a potent drug that you'll take at least three times a day for the rest of your life. Once food is broken down into it's basic components (glucose, amino acids, and fatty acids) and sent into the bloodstream, it has a more powerful impact on your body - and your health — than any drug your doctor could ever prescribe."

Dr. Barry Sears, Ph.D.
Enter The Zone

We all know that eating is a fundamental part of our daily existence. Eating supplies our body with nutrients to produce energy, assist with new tissue building and repair, and enhance the countless metabolic functions within our bodies. Heyer (*A Beginners Introduction to Nutrition*) states that nutrition is a process. It is the interaction between the organisms in the body and their nutrient environment. Heyer also maintains that this interaction represents a series of activities through which body organisms absorb and convert food. This conversion is essential for healthy growth and repair of cells and intercellular materials. Your quality of life and energy levels are dependent upon an adequate dietary supply of nutrients. Nutrients are classified as carbohydrates, proteins, fats, water, vitamins and minerals. These nutrients occur in different combinations and amounts in food. In order to meet our physiological and energy needs for these nutrients, a proper combination of these various foodstuffs must be consumed daily.

However, based on current data, the "American Way" of food consumption may not be the right way. A typical American diet contains over 30 percent of its calories from fat, with about half of the population obtaining up to 40 percent of its calories from this source. In terms of weight, these estimates by health experts could equal up to 100 grams of fat a day. This point was further clarified by Dr. Anthony J. Cichoke, M.A. D.C., an internationally known writer, lecturer, and researcher. Dr. Cichoke maintains that most of us eat too many calories (from empty carbohydrates, salt, sugar, and fat), but not enough complex carbohydrates and other nutrients. In fact, a national survey of over 21,000 people showed that not one American received 100% of the recommended daily allowance for 10 basic nutrients from their diet.

We now know that it is the improper or inadequate consumption of nutrients than not only encourages or perpetuate cycles of chronic fatigue but is the major cause of the collapse of the body's metabolic machinery.

As cited by Dr. Frederick Hatfield and Daniel Gastelu, M.S. authors of *Dynamic Nutrition For Maximum Performance*,

> *Hundreds of diets and other nutritional programs have been created for weight loss, but very few have been designed to promote the maximum amount of biological energy. Formulating a plan that will use a variety of foods to boost the body's "ATP" production capabilities are vital in creating internal conditions which allow the organism to realize its full metabolic energy potential.*

When human bioenergetics and dietary preferences are viewed from this context, it becomes apparent that simply eating and proper nutrition are not one in the same. I firmly believe that you have the ability over your lifetime to escape from exhaustion by adhering to the eight key principles cited below:

Key #1 — Know Your Nutrition
Key #2 — Know Your Correct Calorie Ratio Requirement

Key #3 — Understanding Calorie Ratios
Key #4 — Eat with Awareness
Key #5 — Utilize The Glycemic Index of Foods
Key #6 — Control The Insulin/Glucogen Axis
Key #7 — Practice Proper Food Combining
Key #8 — Recognizing Food Sensitivities

The food you eat helps the body form the cell's "ATP", our main biological energy source. As we have learned, all living things consist of a vast system of cells which grow; function, multiply, die and have to be replaced. All these events not only need the raw materials but also the driving force that ensures their incorporation into a growing entity (namely yourself) and the removal or further utilization of waste product. We need food and we need energy, and the source of both of these is our diet.

In any sound program aimed at assisting the body in its attempts to manufacture biological energy, proper nutritional choices are paramount. In this chapter I will show you how non-adherence to the eight principles just cited, have contributed greatly to the current human energy crisis.

Know Your Nutrition

In physiological terms, food satisfies three fundamental body needs:

1. The need for energy;
2. The need for new tissue and tissue repair;
3. The need for chemical regulations of the metabolic functions constantly taking place in the body.

Human biological needs are provided for by six classes of compounds called nutrients. These six classes are: carbohydrates, fats, proteins, minerals, vitamins, and water. Nutrients are classified as macronutrients or micronutrients. Proteins, carbohydrates, fats, and water, the macronutrients together account for most of the weight of food. Vitamins and minerals, the micronutrients, however, constitute less than one percent of the weight of food. The importance of each category of nutrient is highlighted below:

Carbohydrates

Carbohydrates are the most efficient source of "food energy." Carbohydrates are classified as simple and complex. Complex carbohydrates are generally starches, such as wheat, rice, bread and pasta, which give you a slower sustained release of energy. The "simple carbs" like sucrose, table sugar, are less efficient energy boosters and tend to actually depress energy levels over time. Carbohydrates yield 4 calories of energy per gram.

Fats

Fats are essential in our diets. They are the most concentrated source of food energy, containing twice as many calories per unit as protein or carbohydrates. They are, therefore, a storage form of excess energy. Because of the long-term negative consequences of a high-fat diet, however, we must restrict our intake of fats, particularly saturated fats. Fats yield 9 calories of energy per gram.

Protein

The third source of the six major classes of nutrients is protein. Protein is a major structural component of all body tissue and is needed for growth and repair. In addition, it is a functional component of enzymes, hormones, antibodies, blood plasma, transport mechanisms and a host of other maintenance materials. In general, proteins are an inefficient source of energy and are used for energy only when the more efficient sources, carbohydrates and fats, are not available. Protein yields 4 calories of energy per gram.

Minerals

Mineral nutrients are comprised of two groups, those present in relatively large amounts (macro minerals) in the body and those in very small amounts (the trace minerals).

The first group, all available in the foods we eat, are: sodium, potassium, calcium, phosphorus, magnesium, sulfur, and chloride.

There are at least 14 trace minerals like zinc, manganese, cobalt, chromium, fluorine, iodine and iron which must be ingested by humans for the maintenance of health.

Vitamins

Vitamins are organic substances which function as chemical regulators and are necessary for growth and the maintenance of life. Vitamins help produce the body's energy and serve as the structural components or catalysts for growth and tissue repair.

Water

Water is the most "essential" of all nutrients since it takes priority over all others in the need for a constant and uninterrupted supply. An adequate supply of water is necessary for all energy production in the body. Depriving the body of water absolutely limits energy and endurance.

Although vitamins and minerals supplements are taken daily by millions of Americans, the macronutrients from food are your first line of defense against fatigue. If you want more vitality, vigor and vim, the macronutrients must be given first consideration. Vitamins and minerals in supplement form virtually pass thru the system unabsorbed into the bloodstream without the aid of the macronutrients.

Additionally, the energy capacity of each one of the macronutrients varies.

The Power of Carbohydrates

Carbohydrates are the body's main source of energy for virtually all of its functions. During digestion, glucose (a sugar) which circulates in the bloodstream serves as the body's chief energy source. This blood sugar provides the essential energy for our brain and central nervous system. Carbohydrates also have a regulating influence on protein metabolism. The presence of sufficient carbohydrates to meet energy demands prevents protein utilization for energy purposes. Carbohydrates also modulate fat metabolism as fats need carbohydrates for their conversion or breakdown into fatty-acids within the liver.

According to Dr. Sue Rodwell Williams, Ph.D., R.D., former Chief of Nutrition at the Kaiser-Permanente Medical Center in Oakland California, the amount of carbohydrate stored in the liver, muscle tissue and blood stream is about 365 grams. This 365 grams of carbohydrates (glucose) can provide energy to conduct moderate duties up to 13 hours.

This is why the body needs an infusion of carbohydrates throughout the day to meet this physiological need.

Special Note: The brain totally depends on the glucose from carbohydrate for its survival. Glucose provides the energy for central nervous system activity, as the brain has no stored glucose (called glycogen). Without a steady supply of carbohydrates, severe and traumatic hypoglycemic (low blood sugar) shock can cause irreversible brain damage.

The following guide represents examples of some simple and complex carbohydrates.

SIMPLE CARBOHYDRATES

- BARLEY MALT
- CORN SYRUP
- FRUITS
- FRUIT JUICES
- HONEY
- LACTOSE (MILK SUGAR)
- MAPLE SYRUP
- TABLE FLOUR
- WHITE RICE
- WHITE SUGAR

COMPLEX CARBOHYDRATES

- BROWN RICE
- LEAFY GREEN VEGETABLES
- LEGUMES
- LENTILS
- NAVY BEANS
- OATMEAL
- POTATOES (WHITE AND SWEET)
- VEGETABLES
- WHOLE GRAIN BREADS
- WHOLE GRAIN PASTA

Energy Gained, Energy Lost

There has been and is still much controversy concerning correct carbohydrate intake. While there is no recommended dietary allowance (RDA) now called "reference daily intake" (RDI) for carbohydrates, the National Academy of Sciences suggest a total daily carbohydrate intake of 300 grams. Many nutritionally orientated researchers recommend that 70% of your total calories consumed daily should be from carbohydrates, with 50 to 60% of that total being complex.

I do not recommend that you start out with such a high ratio of carbohydrates. One of the major reasons for your low energy levels is probably due to what scientists refer to as "adrenal exhaustion". The adrenal glands, which are located atop your kidneys, assist your body in handling stress, stabilize your blood sugar levels, modulate metabolism, influence central nervous system activity, as well as control the proper maintenance of several hormonal systems.

Over a lifetime, too much coffee, alcohol, stress, fatty fried and processed foods, arthritis (and other chronic illnesses), white flour, candies and sweets, all stress the adrenals making them work overtime to keep your blood sugar levels balanced and maintain your alertness and energy. Flooding the system with an abundance of carbohydrates too quickly can overburden adrenals that are already working overtime.

We shall cover correct ratios of carbohydrates and the other macronutrients in another section of this chapter. The key is finding a balance that will augment the body's attempt to make biological energy, not override it.

Please Note: Over the last decade there has been a major campaign by health officials to have Americans reduce their consumption of dietary fat. Conversely, there has been an increase in carbohydrate consumption (especially simple carbohydrates). Please remember: carbohydrates, although the body's preferred fuel source, consumed in excess of biological need, are stored as fat, thus causing weight gain and creating conditions that inhibit the proper manufacture of biological energy.

Fats

Fats are the most concentrated source of energy. Fatty deposits in your body not only store energy, but also help insulate your body, as well as support and cushion your organs. Fats also help your body absorb fat-soluble vitamins from your intestines. When oxidized (combined with oxygen), fats furnish more than twice the number of calories per gram furnished by carbohydrates and or proteins. Like carbohydrates, fats are composed of the basic structural elements of carbon, hydrogen and oxygen. Fat has a relatively high hydrogen content therefore making it a much more concentrated form of fuel. However, it has to go through more changes to produce energy, so it is not a "quick" form of energy like carbohydrates. Fats are considered more as a storage form of energy to be utilized as needed by the body.

The major source of energy from fat comes from the fatty acids. Yes, there are fats that are actually good for you in moderation and are critical to human bioenergetics and physiology. Commonly known as "UFA's" (unsaturated fatty acids), these types of fatty acids are found in liquid vegetable oils such as wheat germ, soy, safflower and corn oil. Unsaturated fatty acids assist in the process of cellular-respiration, tissue, and organ oxygenation. As a point of reference, respiration is the entire set of physical and chemical processes involved in the taking in of oxygen and the giving off of carbon dioxide (waste).

Current data suggest that daily fat intake should consist of 65 grams of fat. Of that amount, no more than 20 grams should come from saturated sources. Saturated fats are the hard fats, like butter and other fats that remain solid at room temperature.

Although fats serve as a valuable source of energy, they can pose several problems. Consumed in excess of physiological need, fats cause weight gain, clog your arteries, impede normal metabolic functions, raise blood pressure and elevate harmful cholesterol (LDL) levels. The major source of the problem is overconsumption of saturated fats. Presently, Americans consume over 40% of their daily calories from fat. This means that the average American eats about 100 pounds of fat a year. From a nutritional and bioenergetic standpoint this is excessive and will sap the energy from your existing "energy pool". Consuming this much fat, besides compromising your ability to make biological energy, can jeopardize your health.

To meet physiological needs, 25% of the above total would be sufficient. Due to the above factors, I strongly recommend that you begin adjusting your total fat intake to about 65 grams a day, with at least 50% of that total coming from unsaturated sources. By doing this you can substantially increase the efficiency of your body's metabolic energy potential.

A Fat Primer

To give your system the thrust of power it needs, begin replacing unhealthy saturated fats with essential fatty acids. Essential literally means just that. The human body is incapable of making these fatty acids. They must come from dietary or supplementary sources. Linoleic and linolenic acids are the two essential fatty acids that must come from dietary sources.

The National Research Council maintains that 1% of fat intake should include calories from EFA's. For optimum health, I generally suggest that 3% to 5% of fat intake come from essential fatty acids.

A deficiency of essential fatty acids can lead to improper enzyme function within the cell. This occurrence can hinder energy production and proper metabolism of fats. The need for essential fatty acids increases in proportion to saturated fat consumption and carbohydrate intake. A teaspoon, twice daily, of unsaturated fatty acids will greatly enhance your efforts to skyrocket your energy levels. Use the guide below as you begin to make adjustments to your diet.

Unsaturated Fatty Acids The Good Fats		Saturated Fats The Bad Fats
• Black Currant Oil	• Omega 3's (Fish oil)	• Butter
• Borage Oil	• Primose Oil	• Coconut Oil
• Canola Oil	• Safflower oil	• Hydrogenated Oils (Any types)
• Evening Primrose Oil	• Soy bean Oil	• Lard
• Flax Oil	• Sunflower oil	• Margarine
• Olive Oil	• Wheat Germ Oil	• Palm Oil

Please Note: Fats, no matter what type, consumed in excess of dietary need will only hamper your energy program. Stick to the guidelines as outlined. Unsaturated fatty acids can also be purchased in capsule form in vitamins and health stores.

Protein

In my daily contact with consumers, students, bodybuilders, cyclists, and amateur athletes, I am confronted with the great myth about protein. Many people are still unaware that protein is a poor source of energy. You are essentially a protein being. Your hair, skin, nails, enzymes, blood, immune system, muscles, hormones, and internal organs, including your heart and brain, are all made from the protein you consume.

Protein should be thought of as a back-up fuel source. When inadequate amounts of carbohydrates and fats are present, the body will breakdown existing muscle tissue to meet its physiological needs. When this happens, not only will your energy levels plummet, your metabolic rate (the rate at which your body utilizes calories) will slow down. Pound for pound muscle is the most efficient metabolic agent you have; however, it is an 'expensive' energy source.

Nitrogen Balance

Your overall health and strength will gradually decline if your body stays in what is scientifically known as a "negative nitrogen balance". The body uses nitrogen from protein to help keep it in a growth state.

Besides being the major building material for your internal and external structures, protein, like carbohydrates, provides four calories per gram consumed. These calories serve as sources of heat and energy. By consuming enough carbohydrates and fats, your body can use these calories to help rebuild you and your internal energy blueprint. **This is good!**

The National Academy of Science recommends that you get 50 grams of protein daily. However, protein needs can vary greatly from individual to individual. The National Research Council recommends that .42 grams of protein be consumed daily for each pound of body weight. Dr. Barry Sears, author of the highly acclaimed book *Enter the Zone*, maintains that the most beneficial ratio of protein in relationship to carbohydrate intake is 3 grams of protein to every four grams of carbohydrate; regardless of individual genetics.

Please Note: *One of the biggest misconceptions about protein is that it will not make you fat. Protein consumed in excess of actual need (building new structures and providing energy) will be converted by the liver to fat and stored in body tissue as such.* **This is not healthy. Balance is the key.**

Also, stress greatly increases your need for protein.

Protein is found abundantly in most meats, poultry, eggs, dairy products, as well as fruits, seeds, nuts, legumes and vegetables. The latter are known as incomplete proteins because they do not contain all of the essential amino acids (the building blocks of protein). There are 22 known amino acids. Eight of them (the essential ones) cannot be made by the body and must be provided by dietary or supplemental means.

Special Note: *A high protein meal can raise metabolism about 25% above normal while a high carbohydrate meal boosts metabolism only by about 5%.*

Why Nutritional Needs Differ

The ratio and amounts of nutrients necessary for optimum health is different for each individual person since each of us is biochemically different. You are biochemically unique, and individual, even if you have an identical twin, according to Dr. Jeffrey Bland, a professor of nutritional biochemistry and former director of the Linus Pauling Laboratory of Nutrient Analysis in Palo Alto, California. The weight of your various organs, the activities of the many enzymes within the tissues of your body, the way your nervous system translates messages from the environment into physiology action, and the function of your immune and endocrine (glandular) systems are all unique to you. In order to achieve the highest level of energy and wellness, it is important for you to supply your body with the correct ratio of nutrients, in amounts that will sustain your individual metabolic potential.

In today's environment it also is important to compensate for the external forces that you cannot control, such as poor nutrient content, soil variability, environmental pollutants, pesticides, and genetically altered foods. All of the aforementioned categories increase our biological need for nutrients. This is why many nutritional researchers and environmentalists insist that organically grown foods, pound for pound, supply more energy-rich nutrients.

Internal weaknesses such as depressed immunity, physical and emotional stress, chronic diseases (diabetes, arthritis, heart disease) as well as sluggish eliminative organs (liver, kidneys, colon) all increase the body's need for nutrients. To compensate for these negative internal and external forces, numerous studies of both laboratory animals and humans have shown that eating several mini-meals will fortify and rejuvenate both the body and mind.

These observations lead to several basic dietary questions:
- How much food should I consume daily?
- How many servings of each category do I need?
- What about my individual weaknesses and biochemistry?

Elta Saltos, a nutritionist at the United States Department of Agriculture and Human Nutrition Information Service in Washington D.C., suggests starting with the "Food Guide Pyramid". She maintains that the food pyramid can help put dietary guidelines into action. The food pyramid illustrates food guidelines outlined by the U.S. Department of Agriculture. It is based on the most up-to-date information on food scientific research. Based on this data, nutritional scientists suggest these ranges to maintain optimal health and to meet physiological energy needs. Figure 4.2 (see next page) also list exactly how many servings of each food group you should consume daily.

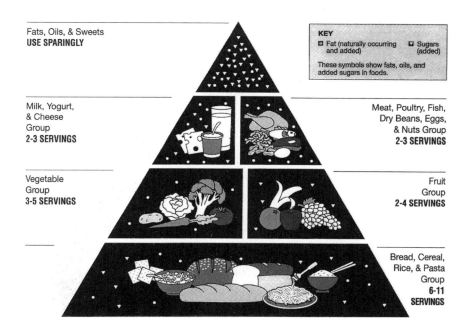

So the question then becomes, if I consume the quantities or servings as stipulated by the U.S. Department of Agriculture, should I be able to increase my energy levels. The answer to that question, is — not necessarily so.

One of the most important aspects of building biological energy nutritionally is understanding the science of calories and food ratios. It is proper timing of nutrient intake in proper proportions that actually brings energy into life!

Know Your Correct Calorie Requirement

Saltman, Gurin and Mothner (1987), state that "the trick to eating nutritiously is to use the RDA's and other recommendations as a guide without turning them into a rigid diet plan." They suggest that you also need to maintain a sensible balance of energy-providing nutrients. For maximum energy output, they advise following the recommendations by the American Heart Association and the National Cancer Institute which are:

- Meet at least 50 percent of your energy needs with carbohydrates but limit intake of refined sugars to only 10 percent. (I however, strongly suggest that you work toward zero intake of refined sugars).
- Take on no more than 35 percent of your calories in fats and only 10 percent in saturated fats.
- Get about 15-20 percent of your calories from protein.
- And, within this balance, take all the vitamins and minerals you need.

One of the major reasons you should not use the recommended dietary allowances as a rigid guide in determining your correct calorie ratio is their generalized nature. RDA's are mainly based on the needs of a person in "perfect health". They don't take into account the intricate necessities of the individual. The key question concerning energy and proper nutrition then becomes, **Are You Eating Enough Food, Your Main Energy Source?**

Understanding Calorie Needs

To maintain more stable energy levels, it is important to know how many calories you need to sustain yourself properly. This refers to the amount of calories you need to:

1. Maintain internal metabolic processes (breathing, circulation, digestion.)
2. Maintain physical and mental activity level (muscular work, combating stress, thinking, having sex)

The FDA and the Food Safety and Inspection Service of the U.S. Department of Agriculture have adopted a baseline of 2,000 calories. They recommend using the baseline to figure your calorie needs for the energy-producing nutrients: carbohydrates, fats and proteins.

In spite of the above, as we have learned, individual calorie needs vary. Some people need more, others less. Among the factors that have to be considered according to Virginia Wilkening, a registered dietician in the FDA's office of Food Labeling, are:

- body size
- age
- height
- weight
- activity
- metabolism

One area you should pay special attention to is activity. What tasks you anticipate completing and the amount of additional food calories needed to accomplish these tasks, without negatively affecting your current energy level is important. The activity levels cited below and accompanying ratios will give you an idea of how to determine your correct calorie intake based on anticipated activity levels.

Very Light: Driving, typing, painting, laboratory work, ironing, sewing, cooking, playing cards, playing a musical instrument, other seated or standing activities.

Light: Housecleaning, child care, garage work, electrical trade work, carpentry, restaurant work, golf, sailing, table tennis, walking on a level surface at 2.5 to 3 miles per hour.

Moderate: Weeding, hoeing, carrying a load, cycling, skiing, tennis, dancing, walking 3.5 to 4 miles per hour.

Heavy: Heavy manual digging, basketball, climbing, football, soccer, carrying a load uphill.

Source: FDA Consumer, Focus on Food Labeling, U.S. Food and Drug Administration, Rockville, MD., May 1993, p.44

To determine your individual calorie requirements, use the formula cited below.

Each of the activity levels listed above will also be used in the formula. For example, very light activity would have a percentage of 20%, light 50%, moderate 70%, and heavy 100%.

Establishing Your Individual Calorie
And Energy Needs

Each of us requires a specific amount of calories at any given moment. Individual needs are based on how many calories you need to maintain the body's internal metabolic processes. This is referred to scientifically as a person's basal metabolism energy need. Overall caloric requirements are based upon the need to maintain basal metabolic activities plus added voluntary activities. Hence the need to assign baseline percentages to activity levels. Basal energy needs are based on our weight in kilograms times the number of hours in a day. To determine your approximate calorie or energy needs:

Step One: Base kilograms for a male is 70kg. Multiply 70kg times 24 (hours in a day) 70x24-1680 calories. This number represents the baseline of calories needed to keep your heart beating, body temperature stable and other metabolic processes going. Please keep in mind that the base kilograms is a general approximation for an adult. To establish your exact base kilogram number based in your weight divide your pounds by 2.2 lbs. Example 200 lbs ÷ 2.2 lbs/kg = 91 kg (kilograms).

Step Two: Now use the percentage established for the type of activity level you will be involved in. Multiply this number by your baseline of calories.

For example:

1680 x .20 = 336 (.20 represents baseline percentage for very light activity.)

This number 336 represents how many additional calories you will need to meet your individual energy requirements based on your anticipated activity level. The three hundred and thirty six additional calories should be added to your baseline number of 1680 which equals 2,016 calories.

This brings us back full circle to the earlier comments by Hatfield and Zucker on why our nutrient intake should be based on what we are going to be doing, not what we just did.

This exercise will allow you to easily determine your correct calorie and energy needs. For women, use the same process; however, your baseline number to start with would be 58kg.

Now that you know how to calculate the exact amount of calories you need to maintain your metabolic energy needs, a key question comes to mind. That question is,

In what proportions or food groups would these calories be the most beneficial?

Understanding Calorie Ratios

Once you have established the number of calories you need throughout the day, you can begin to establish concise dietary goals. Over the past decade there has been a tremendous amount of new information regarding the effect food has on mood, energy levels and even sexual desire. Today, researchers know that certain foods in specific amounts are necessary for optimal health. For example, besides providing us with energy, a good diet should help prevent heart disease, stroke, cancer, and guard against obesity, and its related negative health consequences.

Over the last decade there has been mounting evidence that the intake of certain ratios of various food groups will protect us against a host of diseases, such as cancer, arthritis and diabetes. Conversely, researchers have discovered that certain food groups consumed in certain ratios and at certain times have a profound impact on how we feel and the amount, as well as the duration, of the vitality we experience.

Let's take a look at a few of these ratios and find out why some are more applicable at certain times than others.

The Science Behind The Ratios

If you remember our earlier conversation, your intake of nutrients should be based on what you will be doing for the next several hours, not what you just did. By using the activity level percentages as a guide, you can formulate a nutritional plan of attack based on the proposed activity in front of you. When you see numbers listed like 60-20-20, 70-20-10 or 40-30-30 regarding macronutrient intake, the first number represents the percentage of carbohydrates, the second protein, and the third fat. While there are different suggested available ratios, it is important that you understand these values and the reasoning behind their use.

The most widely advocated diet regimen over the past several years has been the 70-15-15. This ratio represents a high intake of carbohydrates, low protein and low-fat intake. This diet ratio would benefit individuals looking for quick, immediate burst of energy. Current data, however, indicates that a large portion of the American public don't respond well to high-carbohydrate, low-protein, low-fat diets. These individuals are classified as being insulin resistant. In this condition, insulin levels remain high because blood sugar levels do not fall. This due to the fact that certain cells are unresponsive to insulin's transportation into them. This condition is known as "hyperinsulinemia", which can lead to diabetes and heart disease.

Unlocking Your Energy Potential Nutritionally

The above occurrence can be compared to you knocking on the door to your son or daughter's room, to which they usually respond by opening the door. However, in the case of hyperinsulinemia, you knock, there is a response, but the door does not open. When this happens your appetite increases, fat storage accelerates and your metabolism slows down. As a result of these new findings, many health experts today advocate an intake of calories based on a ratio of 40-30-30. Forty percent carbohydrates, 30% protein and 30% fat.

I support this contention, as data indicates that the extra protein will help keep blood sugar levels stabilized and insulin down. This will definitely help reduce the "crash" some people experience when energy levels begin to plummet due to the ingestion of excessive amounts of simple carbohydrates. A balance of nutrients is the key. This ratio of macronutrient intake would allow you to:
- meet physiological energy needs
- replenish glycogen stores (the body needs about 450 gram of carbohydrates daily to replace stored glycogen)
- Provide enough protein for building and maintenance

purposes
- Keep blood sugar levels stabilized
- Stimulate metabolism and refuel Krebs Cycle activities
- Prevent energy crashes (provided 40 to 50% of carbohydrate intake are complex carbohydrates)
- Control your appetite and prevent episodes of binge eating
- Eliminate cravings for sweets
- Prevent ketosis (body's use of fats and proteins to fuel metabolic cycles)

Computing Exact Macronutrient Intake

As you have probably realized, determining which ratio is right for you is not an exact science. In all probability, you will have to discover by trial and error which ratio works best for you. The important thing to remember here is that you can customize a particular ratio to meet your individual needs. Additionally, you can change ratios as your activity level and lifestyle dictates. This fact makes for an exciting challenge and puts you in total control of jump-starting, reaching and realizing your full energy potential.

Figure 4.2 that follows gives a general overview of a few of the most popular diet ratios utilized today. It is important to remember that these ratios can be tailored to meet specific needs, such as preparing for an event, or just to help restore balance.

The Ratios
Figure 4.2

Ratio	Nutrient Content	Major Focus	Advantage	Disadvantage
1.70-15-15 The A-typical Low-protein, Low-fat American Diet	70%-carbs 15%-protein 15%-fat	Glycogen storage quick energy	Supplies fuel to cells and brain great for improving endurance	Can promote increased insulin production which can cause fat storage and may induce cravings for carbs causing binge eating.
2. 80-10-10 The vegetarian Diet	80% carbs 10% protein 10% Fat	same as above	Prevent low blood sugar or hypoglycemia better suited for slow Metabolic types	May not provide adequate amounts of protein and fat to meet known dietary needs. Can cause drowsiness and impair concentration.
3. 60-20-20 American Diabetes diet recommendation	60% carbs 20% protein 20% fat	adequate replenishment of blood sugar and metabolism	provides energy fosters less restriction of calorie intake promotes glycogen production	For some individuals may pose problems in blood sugar stability and dips in energy levels
4. 40-30-30 The New Diet Plan	40% carbs 30% protein 30% fat	balanced nutritional Intake stable, steady burst of energy	less hunger, steady energy glycogen promotion system Repair and steady Metabolic activity.	May be inappropriate for persons with cholesterol and tryglyceride elevation. May not replenish blood glucose or glycogen levels fast enough during high intensity exercise or workout routines. Not well suited for slow metabolic types.

Energy Metabolism and Metabolic Typing

According to Ann Louise Gittleman, M.S., C.N.S., one of America's top nutritionists, determining your metabolic type is the most important step in this whole process. Your individual metabolic rate determines how fast your body will convert the food you consume into fuel. Brenda Garrison, R.D., of the Cooper Wellness Program in Dallas Texas, maintains that there are several ways to test human metabolic activity. Through the use of a device that measures oxygen consumption and carbon dioxide production, scientists can determine a person's metabolic capacity.

To effectively produce biological energy, our bodies must first properly digest the foods we eat, converting carbohydrates into glucose, fats into fatty acids, and proteins into amino acids. This process releases energy which is captured in high-energy bonds between phosphate and the adenosine molecule to form "adenosine tri-phosphate" (ATP). To replace the ATP used by the cell, another much slower chemical process combines carbohydrate, fats, and proteins with oxygen, and uses the energy derived to form new ATP. When stored, ATP (which is utilized quickly, especially while exercising) vanishes, the cells begins to create more "ATP". Scientist refer to this process as "energy metabolism." You might ask:

- How fast does your body convert food to fuel?
- What metabolic type are you?

To get a general idea of your metabolic type, please take the short quizzes on the next page. (Figures 4.3 and 4.4)

Slow-Burner Questionaire

1. Are you somewhat laid-back and even-tempered?   yes ____ no ____
2. Does red meat feel heavy in your system?   yes ____ no ____
3. Do you approach problems one step at a time, rather than juggling many at once?   yes ____ no ____
4. Can you skip breakfast without losing energy or getting hungry?   yes ____ no ____
5. Do sweet things like candy or fruit give you a quick pick-up?   yes ____ no ____
6. Do you prefer a light meal or salad or pasta to a "heavier" one steak and potatoes?   yes ____ no ____
7. Do you get thirsty a lot?
8. Do foods like cheese, butter and avocados seem to make you sluggish? yes ____ no ____
9. Does coffee start your morning off just right?   yes ____ no ____
10. Do you feel you need a pick-up from spices and particularly enjoy tangy condiments like mustard, ketchup and salsa with your food?   yes ____ no ____

If you answered yes to eight or more of these questions, you are a classic slow-burner type and need to target your exercise program to the basic slow-burner regimen?

Fast-Burner Questionaire

1. Do you consider yourself high strung or feel hyperactive? yes ____ no ____
2. Do you actually feel better eating a plate of chops rather than leaner meats like chicken? yes ____ no ____
3. Dp you enjoy a hearty, high-protein breakfast (eggs and bacon)? yes ____ no ____
4. Do you reach for salty snacks like nuts or potato chips when you are stressed out? yes ____ no ____
5. Are avocados, cheesy sauces and full-fat dairy products very satisfying to you? yes ____ no ____
6. Do you feel better eating full meals every two to three hours? yes ____ no ____
7. When you eat sweet foods like cakes and cookies, do you burn out quickly after a short burst of energy?
8. Do you have a hearty appetite? yes ____ no ____
9. Does drinking coffee make you nervous? yes ____ no ____
10. Does a pat of butter on toast satisfy you more than jam? yes ____ no ____

If you answered yes to eight or more of these questions, you are a classic fast-burner type and need to target your exercise program to the basic fast-burner regimen?

Source: Ann Louise Gittleman, *Your Body Knows Best*, Pocket Books, New York, NY., 1996.

What To Do

After you have completed the quizzes, now you can now begin to put all your calculations into practice. You are ready to start determining which foods you should be eating based on your metabolic type. By doing so, you can dramatically increase the efficiency of your body's ability to convert food into usable fuel.

If you are a slow metabolic type, I suggest that you start with a ratio of macronutrient intake in the 60-20-20 or 60-30-10 range. Some foods to consider:

- Proteins — lean beef, chicken (white-meat), turkey
- Grains — brown rice, oatmeal
- Fruits — apples, bananas, cantaloupe, honey dew, oranges, and other citrus fruits
- Fats and oils — olive oil, canola oil, flaxseed oil
- Vegetables — cabbage, carrots, celery, lettuce potatoes, broccoli, beets, cucumbers, kale
- Dairy — Low fat cheese, milk and yogurt.
- Seafood — Tuna, flounder, haddock

Fast Metabolic Types

If you are a fast metabolic type, you are a prime candidate for a ratio of 40-30-30. Fast metabolic types need balance to prevent those "crashes" which can occur when blood sugar levels start fluctuating. Too much 'high test' fuel (carbohydrates) coupled with an inborn tendency toward quick conversion of food to fuel, will cause spurts of intense energy followed by catastrophic bouts of fatigue, sluggishness and a general feeling of malaise.

Fast metabolic types need heavier proteins to slow down their inborn metabolic capacity. Some foods to consider:

- Animal proteins — lean beef, lamb, liver, pork chops, steak
- Dairy — Low fat milk, yogurt and cheese
- Vegetables —beans, green beans, potatoes, yams, spinach, broccoli
- Grains — brown rice, oatmeal
- Fats — peanut, almond, and cashew butter
- Seafood — Flounder, halibut, lobster, sardines, shrimp

By following these guidelines you will be able to stay within your individual "Metabolic Sphere."

The Metabolic Sphere

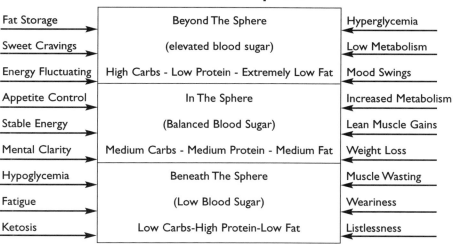

	Beyond The Sphere	
Fat Storage →		← Hyperglycemia
Sweet Cravings →	(elevated blood sugar)	← Low Metabolism
Energy Fluctuating →	High Carbs - Low Protein - Extremely Low Fat	← Mood Swings
	In The Sphere	
Appetite Control →		← Increased Metabolism
Stable Energy →	(Balanced Blood Sugar)	← Lean Muscle Gains
Mental Clarity →	Medium Carbs - Medium Protein - Medium Fat	← Weight Loss
	Beneath The Sphere	
Hypoglycemia →		← Muscle Wasting
Fatigue →	(Low Blood Sugar)	← Weariness
Ketosis →	Low Carbs-High Protein-Low Fat	← Listlessness

Accessing Your Metabolic Sphere

From the above graphic it becomes evident why Dr. Sears contends that food, when broken down into its basic constituents, is powerful medicine. Some foods influence the brain to make substances that calm. Other foods increase the production in the brain of substances that stimulate, energize, and invigorate. The key is knowing which foods initiate 'favorable' responses.

Eat With Awareness

Based on what we have covered thus far, I am confident that you now know that you are primarily a living energy system. Food is the source that fuels all the physiology activities that produce biological energy. The way in which your body utilizes this input of fuel (food) is referred to as "energy metabolism". Different foods, however, have different energy values which food scientists refer to as a kilocalorie. According to the late Nobel Prize-winning chemist, Linus Pauling, the average amount of food energy required by men is 2000 to 3500 kilocalories (Kcal) per day. For women it is 1600 to 2400. He went on to say that young people require more, while older individuals (senior citizens) need less. The average kilocalories needed to satisfy human energy metabolic needs is 2500 kcal. Dr. Pauling states that this amount of energy could heat a bathtub full of water, from 50° F to 100° F. Dr. Pauling went on to say that "if these kilocalories could all be used to do work, they could lift a weight of 1400 pounds to the top of a mile-high mountain."

If food has this type of energy capacity, why is such a large portion of the American public suffering from fatigue. Karen Collins, M.S., R.D., of the American Institute for Cancer Research in Washington, D.C., states that "to keep a more even energy level, don't pack in large amounts of food at one end of the day with relatively little going in at the other". She advises spreading out your meals, throughout the day, not the usual 2 or 3 large meals, but six to eight mini meals. Researchers at the University of Sussex in England also have found that a mid-day 'feast' tends to accentuate the slump most of us hit in the afternoon. In fact, after hearty lunches (in the 1,000 plus calorie range) airplane pilots showed significant losses of visual perception and reaction time, equivalent to missing a night's sleep. When you eat a large meal, the blood vessels supplying the stomach apparently dilate, drawing blood to the gut and away from the brain. When this happens, your energy levels will plummet.

The Food Mood Energy Connection

Is it really possible to impair the body's metabolic energy potential because of what and when we eat? According to Robert Hass, author of *Eat To Win*, and America's top sports nutritionist, the answer is yes! Dr. Judith Wurtman, Ph.D., the distinguished research scientist at M.I.T. (Massachusetts Institute of Technology), states that "you can manage your mood, boost your mental capabilities, and maximize your performance easily and almost instantly by eating foods that have the desired effect on the chemistry of your brain."

Scientists are now exploring how certain nutrients can leave you feeling highly energized. In ground-breaking studies, scientists at M.I.T. looked at how food affects mood. Dr. Wurtman and her colleagues demonstrated that levels of neurotransmitters in the brain could be significantly influenced by the nutrient composition of a single meal. Previously, scientists had thought this was automatically controlled by the brain. The three chemical neurotransmitters: dopamine; norepinephrine; and serotin all have a powerful effect on our mood and energy level.

Dopamine stimulates alertness, and excitement. Norepinephrine is the primary neurotransmitter used by the sympathetic nervous system that stimulates alertness. Researchers at M.I.T. discovered that:

- A protein rich meal can raise levels of norepinephrine and dopamine increasing alertness and assertiveness.
- A meal rich in carbohydrates and low in proteins will increase serotin levels, inducing a relaxed or even sleepy state.

If you eat protein, either alone or with a carbohydrate and your brain is rapidly using up its supply of dopamine or norepinephrine, it will use tyrosine supplied by the protein to manufacture more of these neurotransmitters. When that happens, you'll find yourself more alert, more motivated, more mentally energetic and "up".

If, on the other hand, you eat "carbohydrates alone, without protein," more tryptophan (a protein amino acid) will be made available to your brain which will use it to make more serotonin.

As a result, you will feel less stressed, less anxious, more focused and relaxed.

This phenomenon explains why eating cacao and chocolate have become daily rituals for some. They both contain an amino acid that stimulate neurotransmitters that affect mood, sexual desire and libido.

To test and measure your sensitivity to proteins and carbohydrates at various times of the day, use the following guide formulated by Dr. Wurtman. The test can be conducted at breakfast, lunch and dinner, using various carbohydrate and protein combinations.

Guidelines

1. No more than fifteen minutes before each test meal or snack, rate your mood or state of mind at that moment. Do it by placing 0, 1 or 2 next to each descriptive word in the before meal column of the questionnaire. Use 0 for adjectives that do not apply, 1 for those that apply only slightly, and 2 when the feeling is intense.
2. An hour after your meal or snack, rate your state of mind again in the "after meal" column of the questionnaire.

Food-Mood Questionnaire

State of Mind	Before Meal	After Meal
Alert		
Energetic		
Relaxed		
Calm		
Irritable		
Tense		
Sluggish		
Sleepy		
Sad		
Despairing		

Interpreting Your Test Scores

If your score sheets show many changes from 0 to 2 or 2 to 0 in your before and after meal state of mind, your food can be a potent tool in your attempts to enhance your energy levels.

If your score sheet shows few leaps from 0 to 2 or 2 to 0, but many smaller movements of a lesser degree (say from 0 to 1 or 1 to 0), you are somewhat less sensitive to the food/mind/mood response. For you, learning to take advantage of the mind and mood capabilities of protein and carbohydrates can still make a big difference in your quest.

Why You Should Eat a Good Breakfast

Dr. Wurtman insists that all her clients start every day with a good breakfast. She strongly suggests that you do the same if you want to function in top form from the time you wake until the time you turn out the lights at night. Here's why:

> Getting food into your system in the morning is "entraining." (Entraining is a technical term referring to the support and enhancement of biological processes through synchronization.) Eating at a time when your body is switching from the lower energy expenditures, lower temperatures, and lower hormone production in the nighttime hours into its more active daytime mode helps make these transitions occur more smoothly and efficiently — and with better results for you. When supplied with the proper nutrients and energy just as circadian rhythms are about to peak, your body is a little like a runner with wind at his or her back — effortlessly able to go a little faster and a little farther than otherwise.

The biological energy potential of this timing sequence of nutrient intake can be dramatically enhanced, based on type of food consumed. This basic concept is what nutritional scientists refer to as the "glycemic index of foods." The glycemic index reflects the rate of digestion and absorption of carbohydrates, and how fast it converts to fuel. Knowing how to utilize this natural process will enable you to decide whether you want an immediate or steady rise in the blood sugar.

Knowing how to utilize the food index can blast your energy levels to new heights!

The Glycemic Index of Foods

The major focus of the Glycemic Index concerns a numbering system and how particular foods, based on their assigned numbers, elicit a response. Foods that rapidly raise blood-glucose levels have a high glycemic index number. Those that cause a much slower rise in blood glucose (sugar) levels have a low Glycemic Index (GI) number. Figure 4 which follows gives a breakdown of certain food groups and cites their corresponding GI number. If you follow the sequence of numbers you will find that the food stuffs with lower numbers are actually better suited for sustained, controlled, and balanced metabolic activities. The higher number foods cause quick release of food energy.

Understanding and utilizing the Glycemic Index can go a long way in controlling how well the body converts food to energy. Health officials contend that consuming those groups of foods which cause a slower rise in blood glucose levels will help you:

- Maintain more stable energy levels throughout the day
- Keep blood sugar levels stabilized
- Prevent binge eating, thus controlling appetite
- Elevate your mood, making you feel more alert
- Encourage lipolysis (the breakdown and utilization of stored fat as fuel)
- Stimulate glycogenolysis (converting stored blood sugar called glycogen into usable glucose)

High glycemic	Moderate glycemic	Low glycemic

Beverages
Gatorade–91
Carbonated soft
  drink–68
**Bread and grain
  products**
Bagel–72
Bread, white–70
Bread, whole wheat–69
Corn flakes–84
Oatmeal–61
Graham crackers–74
Grape Nuts–67
Fruits
Watermelon–72
Raisins–64
Honey–73**
Vegetables
Potato, baked–85
Potato, microwaved–82
	**Bread and grain
	  products**
	Pasta–41
	Rice, white–56
	Rice brown–55
	Pumpernickel bread–41
	Bran muffin–60
	Popcorn–55
	Fruits
	Orange juice–57
	Bananas, overripe–52
	Orange–43
	Apple juice,
	  unsweetened–41
	Vegetables
	Corn–55
	Peas–48
	Sweet Potato–54
	Legumes
	Baked beans–48
	Lentil soup–44
		Fruits
		Apple–36
		Apricots, dried–31
		Bananas, underripe–30
		Grapefruit–25
		Pear–36
		Fructose–23**
		Legumes
		Lima beans–32
		Chickpeas–33
		Green beans–30
		Kidney beans–27
		Lentils–29
		Split peas, yellow–32
		Dairy Products
		Chocolate milk–34
		Skim milk–32
		Whole milk–27
		Yogurt, low-fat, fruit–33
		**Bread and grain
		  products**
		Barley–25
		Power bar–30-35
		PR bar–33

*Index based on 50 grams of carbohydrate per serving.

Figure 4 Source: Susan M. Kleiner, Ph.D., R.D., *Power Eating, Human Kinetics,* Champaign, IL., 1998, p. 50

The chart that follows gives some examples of foods and their specific glycemic index ratings.

SOME USEFUL GLYCEMIC INDEX RATINGS

GLUCOSE	**100**
Baked potato	98
Carrots	92
Honey	87
Cornflakes	80
White Rice	72
Wheat Bread	72
White Potato	70
White Bread	69
Brown Rice	66
Banana	62
SUCROSE	**59**
Yam	51
Spaghetti	50
Orange Juice	46
Grapes	45
Golden Apples	39
Yogurt	36
Ice Cream	36
Whole Milk	34
Skim Milk	32
Peach	29
Grapefruit	26
Cherries	23
FRUCTOSE	**20**

The Insulin / Glycogen Axis

One of the most powerful hormones in your body that you have is insulin. Most of us are familiar with insulin, because it is the stuff many of our relatives take to control their blood sugar. When insulin levels get too high or too low, havoc is wreaked on energy levels. Insulin is produced by the pancreas (a long gland that lies just below the stomach). It is secreted into the bloodstream where it binds to certain proteins known as carriers. The carriers transport insulin into muscle, liver and other tissues for use. Its main job, however, is to regulate blood glucose (sugar) levels, by acting as an intermediary in the metabolism of sugars, carbohydrates, fats and proteins.

The Glycogen Story

During the process of energy metabolism, your body turns food into usable energy to fuel life's processes. The body has the capacity to build a reserve of this energy extracted from food. This free energy pool is known as "glycogen." Glycogen is manufactured as a direct result of carbohydrate metabolism. Glycogen is stored in the liver and in muscle tissue and is called upon when insufficient amounts of macronutrients are consumed.

There is (when nutritional requirements are met) a 12 to 48 hour reserve of glycogen (which is broken down from glucose) available. Because of the body's constant need for energy, glycogen stores can be depleted rapidly. Replenishing glycogen requires an input of food. Non-replenishment of glycogen could be compared to riding around on empty in your automobile, experiencing knocks, pings, poor acceleration, and a feeling of power loss and diminished performance. Athletes call this phenomenon "hitting the wall". As muscle glycogen reserves begin to vanish, so does your intestinal fortitude. It is in this context that the legendary coach of the Green Bay Packers Vince Lombardi's comment becomes applicable. He stated that:

"Fatigue makes cowards of us all"

According to Nancy Clark, M.S., R.D., and author of the *Sports Nutrition Guide Book: Eating to Fuel Your Active Life Style,* despite adequate muscle glycogen, uncoordination, light-headedness, feelings of weakness and inability to concentrate often occur because the liver does not have enough glycogen reserve to fuel the brain. Ms. Clark went on to say that the average 150-pound active male has about 1,800 calories of carbohydrates stored in his liver, muscles and blood in the following quantities:

Muscle glycogen	1,400 calories
Liver glycogen	320 calories
Blood glucose	80 calories
Total	1800 calories

When you do not replenish these stores via-proper macronutrient intake, a "crash" or sudden feeling that your energy has vanished may occur.

Your body utilizes ATP, circulating glucose, glycogen and fat, to produce energy. The major difference in these energy sources is how fast they can release their energy. Glycogen is an important catalyst, as is glucose and fat, in producing biological energy, because they provide the energy for the recycling of, or the manufacture of, "ATP".

Glycogen promotes the movement or utilization of fuel, rather than its storage as insulin does. Glycogen's main job is to raise blood sugar when it gets too low. For example glycogen is responsible for converting protein into a usable fuel, namely glucose. This process is known as gluconeogenesis and occurs in the liver.

Insulin, as previously cited, lowers blood sugar when it gets too high. Using the glycemic index to manipulate or stabilize this hormonal balancing act is crucial to sustaining stable levels of energy. The sources used to balance this Insulin/Glycogen Axis are the basic macronutrients in the diet: carbohydrates, proteins and fats. It is protein, however, that plays a major role in helping to regulate this balancing act. In fact, protein is the macronutrient responsible for the release of both glycogen and to a much smaller degree insulin. It is the carbohydrates that signal the body to circulate insulin into the bloodstream. When these two hormones are working internally, the body's energy levels skyrocket. Concentration increases, heightened awareness occurs as well as a general feeling of wellness. Let's take a closer look at the function of these two hormones and the key role they play in energy metabolism. (Please see next page.)

INSULIN

- Lowers Elevated Blood Sugar

• Shifts metabolism into storage mode	• Changes Glucose and protein into fat
• Encourages Fat storage	• Accelerates cholesterol production
• Promotes Edema (water rention)	• Modulates glucose and its conversion to energy
• Removes glucose from bloodstream to muscles	• Locks up potential stored glycogen
• Shuttles fat into cells	• Can promote diabetes and heart disease in cases of constant elevation

Utilizes Fat and Tissues as energy sources	**GLYCOGEN**	Fuel For Brain

- Encourages body to use fat as a fuel source
- Reduces cholesterol levels
- Elevates low blood sugar levels
- Acts as a diuretic
- Transforms fat and protein to blood sugar
- Boost metabolism
- Increases energy
- Helps restore or recycle ATP

The two most important factors involved with maintaining balance between these two powerful hormones are:

1. The size of the meal you eat.
2. The ratio of protein to carbohydrates. (favorable ratio 3 parts protein to 4 parts carbohydrates)

Those excess calories you have been consuming will continuously keep your insulin levels elevated. This is not healthy! You need to ensure that you are consuming some proteins with those large carbohydrate meals, which brings us back to the balanced 40-30-30 ratio.

Please Note: There is evidence that eating protein rich foods need not be simultaneous with the consumption of carbohydrate-rich foods. This is due to the fact that there is about a "seventeen" hour window in which to balance the two properly.

Based on current data and the nutritional patterns, habits, and preference of Americans, I do not recommend that you attempt to manipulate this so-called window of opportunity. The easiest and least problematic way to modulate the "Insulin/Glycogen Axis" would occur via timing your nutrient intake several times a day (4 to 5), consuming moderate amounts of various macronutrients and micronutrients.

The key, however, is moderation. This will help facilitate digestion and, by adhering to the principle of balanced nutrient intake, will unleash the full metabolic potential and power of those dormant recesses of energy. It is the proper input of nutrients that helps keep your energy system in shape. Proper nutrition is truly nature's key that creates cycles of interminable energy!

Practice Proper Food Combining

Most of the basic rules of food combining break with traditional American eating habits. Many people mistakenly believe that food combining means choosing the right combination of foods to provide complete protein. *More accurately, it is eating foods in combinations that permit easier and more complete digestion.*

Mattson, in reference to food combining, recommends that:

- Fruits in general should be eaten on an empty stomach.
- Proteins and starches generally should not be eaten together, for example, a steak and a baked potato.
- Proteins and starches individually mix well with vegetables.
- Sweet fruits and starches are a poor mix.
- When combining fruits, acid and sub-acid fruits take one to one half hour to digest while sweet fruits take three to four hours.

Wilson (1994) also suggested that the following combinations make great meals:

- Fruits with celery and/or lettuce
- Salad and vegetables with your choice of starch, protein or legumes.
- Salad and vegetables with proteins
- Acid fruit, lettuce or celery with avocado
- Melon with acid fruits
- Baked potato with avocado and vegetables
- Sweet fruit salads or shakes

Dr. Douglas Graham, author of the *High Energy Diet Recipe Guide*, states that the key to good nutrition is "diversity." However, he reminds us that the key to good food combining is "simplicity." The fewer foods eaten at a meal, the better.

Depleting Your Energy Stores With Food

"For starters, proper food combining is the easiest and most profound way to improve digestion — a crucial ingredient for health," says Graham. "Digestion is a most demanding activity, requiring up to 50 percent of the body's energy." Bombarding the system with food combinations that challenge the digestive tract makes digestion more difficult and leads to digestive disorders. Besides painful stomach and intestinal problems, poor digestion leaves little energy for other vital bodily functions.

Although food combining takes thought, by eating more simply and combining only a few foods at each meal, these challenges will be minimized. Most importantly, this process should be fun and appetizing. You are in control of your food choices. For many people, any perceived inconvenience is offset by "immediate" improvements in health, "elevated" energy levels and freedom from digestive distress. Long-term bonuses include permanent weight control, renewed vitality, better endurance and an overall sense of well-being.

Recognizing Food Sensitivity

You should be aware of your own individual food sensitivity. By looking at various food frequencies in your diet, you may be able to spot certain foods that may be causing periods of indigestion, intestinal problems, gas and bloating — all "energy zappers".

Ask yourself whether you are eating well-balanced selections from the major food groups and whether these foods are unprocessed or highly processed. How do you feel after you eat? Are you sleepy, confused, shaky or weak? If so, the foods you are consuming may not be optimal for your individual biochemical needs. Does your diet contain adequate fiber? Do you consume enough fluids to maintain proper intestinal regularity? Do you have intestinal or stomach pain after eating, which may indicate too high a fat level in your diet? Do you have undigested food in your stool, indicating that you are not properly digesting and assimilating your food? According to your responses, you may begin to construct a diet that better meets your needs and matches your biochemical individuality.

To accomplish the above, I suggest that you start a daily food diary for about 30 days. Eat as you normally do — same times, same intervals — also consuming the types and quantities of food you normally consume. Record your responses as indicated above. It is important to know your sensitivity to specific foods. Having allergic reactions and poorly digested foods will impede your body's ability to properly metabolize these foods. Reduced power and vitality will result if these foods begin to hinder or slow down normal channels of elimination.

Putting It All Together

This brings us to a close of chapter four. It is important to remember that the key to improving your energy levels nutritionally is balance. To get started, you should:

1. Learn as much as you can about macronutrients and their role in energy production.
2. Calculate your individual requirement of calories needed per day and divide that number by the number of meals you will be consuming each day.
3. Decide what your nutritional needs will be. For example are you in a race during the next few weeks or are you concerned

with stabilizing blood sugar and/or controlling your appetite, and/or building an overall maintenance and rejuvenation program? *Choose which ratio program is best suited to your needs and allocate your calorie intake accordingly.*

4. Study the attributes of the glycemic index and use it to address immediate energy planning.
5. Start a food diary and record your reactions to certain foods. Eliminate and rotate other foods that are more appropriate.
6. Practice food combining techniques and increase your awareness of digestive problems.
7. Begin to eat with awareness based on your metabolic type.
8. Know your nutrition. Look for ways to expand on your present knowledge. Consider incorporating organic foods, soy, and phytonutrients into your current dietary regimen. Play the rainbow game — rotate the bright, colored fruits and vegetables as replacements for snacks with little or no nutritional value.

Please see Appendix A "A Few Quick Energy Recipes" found in the rear of this book. These recipes will give you an idea how you can use certain food combinations to boost those sagging energy levels.

Conclusions

By now, I am confident that you realize that you are a living energy system with the potential to convert outside sources of energy into life processes. This process is stated by Robyn Landis, author of *Herbal Defense was Meant to be a Simple Process:* give the body all of what it needs and little of what it doesn't and the body will run itself. Scientists have refined this simple concept in their efforts to learn how the body makes use of food energy and its consequent transformation into usable fuel. By mastering the intricacies of the eight keys cited in this chapter, you can continuously unlock, control, and ultimately realize your full energy potential.

Nature has provided all the tools necessary to repeat this endless cycle of energy conversions. To enjoy or reap the benefits of this process, you are going to have to work hard on mastering the food concepts outlined here, but more importantly, the consistent application of these is critical to you attaining the vibrant, youthful, and energetic existence you deserve.

Once you have aligned your nutritional efforts with those of nature's natural metabolic cycles, you can overcome your fatigue, become functionally stronger and maintain peak vitality every day of your life! As stated by the late Dr. Paavo Airola, Ph.D., N.D., once considered to be one of America's foremost nutritionists and the world's leading exponent of "biological medicine":

> *Nutrients are what the human body has to work with in building and maintaining healthy cells, tissues, glands and organs. There is not an action in the body, be it enzymatic, metabolic, hormonal, mental, nervous, physical or chemical that does not require specific nutrients for its performance.*

> *All other modalities, be it drugs, surgery, manipulations, acupuncture, hydro-electro-magneto-therapy, you name it! — can be useful, but they will fail in most cases unless the corrective and supportive nutritional therapy is given priority.*

Keeping Your Energy System In Shape

The input of energy (food) plays a key role in stoking the metabolic processes. However, the body may need some help in realizing its full energy potential. Without a catalyst (something which initiates an action), this natural cycle can be unresponsive, regardless of the input of fuel.

In the next chapter, "Natural Energizers" we will take a look at some of the most widely used natural supplements that assist healty metabolic cycles versus overriding them. These supplements are excellent adjuncts to any sound nutritional program.

Chapter Five

NATURAL ENERGIZERS

"Metabolic enhancers are substances that improve the performance of existing biochemical pathways by providing cofactors, catalysts and substrates (spare parts). These elements support the actions of the system without causing undue stress to its natural actions."

Dr. Konrad Krail, N.D.
Former President of the American
Association of Naturopathic Physicians

According to Dr. Konrad Krail, N.D., 18% of the American population over the age of ten drink coffee. Dr. Krail maintains that coffee is our most popular stimulant. However, although stimulants can create a temporary sense of well-being, energy and exhilaration, they tax metabolic systems and eventually accelerate their demise. He goes on to say that if you classify stimulants according to their strength, that is their ability to change a process or system based on a per unit dose, this increasing strength is usually accompanied by increases in toxicity and/or abuse potential.

Dr. Krail insists that it is important to remember that:

"Stimulants drive a system and may push it beyond its capabilities to perform."

Since most drug stimulants are highly addictive and even natural stimulants can cause dependency, this suggests that long-term use of stimulants is not advisable. Substances taken to reduce or eliminate fatigue are generally classified as:

- Stimulants
- Adaptogens, or
- Metabolic Enhancers

Stimulants, Adaptogens and Metabolic Enhancers

Stimulants are substances that increase the activity of a system. An adaptogen is defined as a substance that increases all-around resistance and can strengthen the entire body. A metabolic enhancer is a substance, element or compound that has the ability to work with established, in-born metabolic processes. In essence, metabolic enhancers work with the body and do not override its natural processes.

To get the long-term results you seek in building and maintaining your energy potential, it would be wise to stick with those supplements that are adaptogenic or serve as metabolic enhancers versus pure stimulants.

A Move Toward Natural Energizers

In 1993, the medical community was stunned by a study that appeared in the *New England Journal of Medicine*. This survey, known as the "Eisenberg Report", clearly showed that a "changing of the guard" from drug therapy to natural alternatives, although silent, has occurred and is spreading into mainstream society. In fact, the above report revealed that one out or every three Americans had used natural therapies to the tune of about $13.7 billion per year!

Amidst growing concerns of the negative and possible long-term adverse affects of prescription drugs, Americans are seeking more natural ways to combat and prevent an array of health problems.

This new trend also has spread to other countries as well. As cited by a recent article in the *Daily Telegraph*, a London based newspaper, almost 75% of the population in Britain use some form of alternative medicine.

Drugs Versus Natural Alternatives

The controversy surrounding the use of natural alternatives has become a complicated matter due to its spread into mainstream society. While these natural alternatives have a long history of use (in many cases, over 5,000 years) their integration into mainstream medicine has only recently begun to occur. Once considered underground alternatives, these natural substances are now being considered as acceptable health options.

The problem with conventional medicine, however, goes a little deeper than this. On average, it costs over $231 million to bring a new drug to the market place. Companies that manufacture drugs are awarded the exclusive rights to market newly approved medicines for 17 years. In essence, that drug company has the power to charge any price they wish during that period. No person, company or other drug manufacturer can create a genuine copy of the drug for that same seventeen-year period.

This, however, is not the case with natural substances. No one can patent chlorophyll, H_2O (water), ginseng, bee pollen, pyruvate, carbohydrates, amino acids or spirulina. All of these substances occur generously in nature and have the ability to assist the body in producing energy.

The Problem With Drugs

Researchers today insist that America is one of the most medicated societies in the world. Also, public concern has grown with drugs like Viagra (the potency pill), Duract (the arthritis pill) and Fen-phen (the diet pill), all of which have mild to serious side affects and have been linked to causing several deaths. The problem with these drugs is the fact that they provided short-term relief for potential problems that may require long-term lifestyle changes. Because of the above consequences, many health officials today insist that prevention of non-life threatening chronic diseases or metabolic disorders is the key, not drugs that tend to override the system, disrupting normal metabolic processes. This is also evidenced by the recent reports concerning the rise in prescription drug overdoses and the consequent movement of the population toward safer alternatives. Furthermore, in response to public pressure, the National Institute of Health (NIH) Office of Alternative Medicine (formed in 1992) was recently allocated millions of dollars in grants to research just how plants and natural supplements augment natural metabolic cycles.

A Long History of Use

Beyond public pressure in the U.S. supporting further research into the efficacy of natural supplements, many of these substances already have a long history of safe, effective use. It is important to remember that what we (Americans) consider to be alternative are, in many parts of the world, the primary form of health care. This is very evident in many parts of Europe, Asia, Japan and China, especially regarding supplementation versus drug usage.

Questions About Natural Energizers

- What are natural metabolic enhancers?
- How do they serve as co-factors to the human bioenergetic process?
- Which ones are most effective?
- How do I take them and how often?
- Can they be used in conjunction with any medications I am presently taking?
- Do I need a prescription for them?
- How long before I should expect results?
- Can I take more than one?
- What side affects should I expect to experience, if any?
- Can I suddenly stop taking these supplements at any time?

Answering these and other questions concerning the efficacy of the array of natural energizers that are available today is the focus of this chapter. Although, as stated previously, many of these "metabolic enhancers" have a long history of safe use, a large percentage of the American population remains unaware of their individual attributes.

My overall goal in this chapter is to educate you on the safety and effectiveness of some of the most well-known natural energizers. To take an in-depth look at the many different types and categories of "natural energizers", this chapter is divided into seven different sections. They are:

1. Accessory Nutrients
2. Amino Acids
3. Herbs
4. Enzymes
5. Vitamins and Minerals
6. Whole Food Factors
7. Emerging Energizers

Accessory Nutrients

"On the basis of an individual's unique genetic nature, a non-essential nutrient may become an essential nutrient for some people who do not have adequate ability to manufacture them within their own bodies. This is called the justification theory."

Dr. Jeffrey Bland, Ph.D.
Professor of Nutritional Biochemistry

Current knowledge of nutritional need has labeled certain nutrients as 'non-essential'. These are classified as non-essential based on the fact that the body can manufacture its own supply of them. Those nutrients labeled as essential are so categorized because the body is unable to make them. These essential nutrients have to be supplied via dietary intake.

However, as expressed by Dr. Jeffrey Bland, a well-known nutritional biochemist, because of certain biochemical factors, some individuals may produce these non-essential nutrients in insufficient quantities to meet their body's needs. Coined the "justification theory", this concept supports the use of certain accessory or non-essential nutritional supplements and or food factors that augment the body's natural attempt to produce them.

This concept has been embraced by health officials today as concerns mount regarding to the number of individuals who suffer from bouts of unexplained systematic fatigue. There are a number or accessories or non-essential nutrients that have a direct bearing on human bioenergetics. This section will review a few of them.

Alpha-lipoic Acid

According to Dr. Dallas Clouatre, Ph.D., a nutritional researcher and author, many "erogogenic" (performance enhancing) products put performance before health in their design. Alpha-lipoic acid, however, is one supplement that actually improves both.

Alpha-lipoic acid is classified as a member of the "vitamin B" family and is known as the metabolic or all-body antioxidant. This is due to the fact that lipoic acid not only acts as a free radical scavenger, it actually "charges" other antioxidants, thus restoring their power, as confirmed in studies by Dr. Lester Packer, the country's leading antioxidant researcher. In other words, lipoic acid can prevent other antioxidants, like vitamin C and E, from being completely oxidized (used up), thus bringing them back to their active state. The other extraordinary thing about this free radical scavenger is that its acts as both a water and fat-soluble nutrient, having the ability to enter all body systems, which is not the case with all antioxidants. Since free radical aggression has been implicated as a causative factor in poor metabolic functions, and vitamins C and E are normally destroyed in the oxidative process of neutralizing free radical aggression, it is important to find a source of "antioxidant regeneration".This is why lipoic acid is considered to be the 'universal' antioxidant. In addition to regenerating vitamins C and E and other antioxidant systems, it also regenerates the actions of CoQ10, the primary molecule used to produce our cellular energy and ATP.

Alpha-lipoic Acid in Action

As food goes through its breakdown process, Alpha-lipoic acid is responsible for converting food, carbohydrates (our main fuel source) and fats into glucose (blood sugar). Once these nutrients are oxidized (combined with oxygen) they must be acted upon by alpha-lipoic acid before continuing into the "Krebs Cycle". As we learned in Chapters Two and Three, once food is broken down into its smaller component parts glucose (carbohydrates), amino acids (protein), and fatty acids (fats) — they enter the Krebs Cycle to be converted into chemical energy (energy for cellular use).

According to Dr. Jim Clark, a biochemical expert for the Henkel Corporation, alpha-lipoic acid is a very important nutrient. A shortage of alpha-lipoic acid would cause a metabolic "traffic jam" and slow down the production process in which energy generated by our digestion of food is captured by the body to form ATP, our energy molecule.

Additional Benefits of Lipoic Acid

- Moves glucose into the cells, thus controlling insulin activity (**Note:** insulin is the most prevalent hormone and most active in the maintenance of energy levels.)
- Used to treat heavy metal poisoning.
  (**Note:** heavy metal accumulation has been linked to the cause of arthritis, Alzheimer's disease, behavioral disorders, attention deficit disorders, chronic fatigue, and a host of other metabolic disorders.)
- Speeds up recovery time from workouts.
- Prevents hardening of the arteries.
- Used in Germany as a treatment for diabetics.

Dosage and Toxicity

Suggested dosage is 50 to 100mg (milligrams) daily. Do not exceed these ranges as large dosages my cause hypoglycemia (low blood sugar), thus having a negative affect on energy levels. Toxic dosages have been noted in long-term animal studies in the range of 400 to 500 mg/kg of body weight per day, equal to approximately 27-34 grams per 150 pounds of human body weight.

Food Sources

Alpha Lipoic Acid is found in appreciable amounts in a variety of foods.

Coenzyme Q10 (Ubiquinone)

As we learned in Chapter One, our energy level and sense of well-being is directly related to how well our cells are utilizing nutrients. In essence, without the energy our cells (some 60 trillion) need, they are unable to keep life's processes going. When the cell can't make enough "ATP", our energy levels begin to plummet and we begin to feel sluggish, lethargic and just plain tired. One nutrient that plays a key role in the breakdown of food and is intimately involved with the accumulation of ATP is Coenzyme Q10, CoQ10 for short.

CoQ10 is similar in structure to vitamin K and E and is found everywhere in the body. Because this compound is so ubiquitous (meaning found everywhere), it was first named "Ubiquinone". First discovered in 1957 and pioneered here in the U.S. by Dr. Karl Folkers, Ph.D., of the University of Texas, CoQ10 is thought of as the controlling agent that produces 95% of all cellular energy.In fact, studies have confirmed that CoQ10 plays a major role in pumping protons across the "mitochondria" membrane. How important is this action? Well without this vital process, your body would not be able to manufacture enough energy to stay alive!

Mitochondria Function

As previously cited, the mitochondria are the tiny powerhouses in the cell that convert food into energy. It is here that the energy produced in each cell of the body is used to repair or make up the tissues and organs of the body.

CoQ10 molecules move between the bioenergy enzymes acting as a "traffic cop", transporting energy from one enzyme into another to create "ATP", which is the chief energy molecule for all living organisms.

Food Source

CoQ10 is found in beef hearts, chicken hearts, sardines, salmon, peanuts and spinach.

Creatine

Creatine is one of the most popular supplements on the market today. Creatine users report increased workout capacity and better recovery from physical routines, while heavy weight resistance trainers have cited increased muscle growth. Like CoQ10, Creatine is intimately involved with "ATP" (adenosine-tri-phosphate) production and, as such, plays a vital role in our natural energy cycles. It is not an anabolic steroid, but is manufactured in the liver as well as in the pancreas and kidney. Creatine is actually made from the amino acids (proteins) arginine, methionine and glycine.

The reason Creatine is thought of as being an anabolic steroid is because of recent clinical studies, as well as anecdotal (word of mouth) testimonials, that show it can accelerate protein synthesis. That is, it helps the body better use protein for building purposes.

However, Creatine's main function is to supply the energy that assists in muscular contraction so that our bodies can do physical work. While Creatine is mainly derived from red meat, blood levels of this non-essential accessory nutrient can change or diminish due to a number of factors, one being a reduction in muscle mass, and another, increasing age.

Additional Benefits of Creatine

- Increases glycogen (stored glucose) utilization.
- Helps shuttle nutrients and water into cells at faster rates.
- Slows down protein breakdown and catabolism (the body breaking down its own muscle to meet energy and building needs.)
- Helps lower blood triglycerides and cholesterol levels (elevated levels are strong negative factors in causing coronary heart disease).

Dosage and Toxicity

For general therapy — 1 to 5 grams daily

For body building purposes —5 grams of creatine 4 times a day for 4 to 5 days (this is known as the creatine load). After load, 5 grams a day, which equals one maintenance dose.

SPECIAL NOTE: *Since creatine is responsible for recycling ADP (adenosine diphosphate) back to ATP to make more energy, demand for building can outpace production. Researchers have found that by going through the loading phase, a significant increase in total creatine present in muscle tissue was observed, up to 50% in some cases. Creatine works best when "spiked" with a carbohydrate drink or fruit juice.*

No known toxic effects have resulted from creatine usage except mild dehydration and occasional gastric upset or intolerance by some individuals. It is great for athletes, older adults and those with active lifestyles. Because of possible dehydration problems for some individuals, drink plenty of fluids when using creatine.

Food Sources

Creatine is most abundant in red meat and the skeletal muscles of animals. Fish, cod, chicken, pork, salmon, tuna, and turkey all contain appreciable amounts of creatine.

NADA (Nicotinamide Adenine Dinucleotide)

NADA is fast becoming the energizer of choice for many Americans This product was made famous by Dr. George D. Birkmayer, M.D., Ph.D, a biochemical researcher. NADA is marketed under trade name "Enada" and can be purchased in health and vitamin stores.

NADA is referred to as coenzyme 1 and is the coenzyme form of the B-vitamin niacin. NADA naturally occurs in all living cells and also contributes to the internal workings of human bioenergetic pathways, especially in the brain and nervous systems.

Research has confirmed that NADA can naturally increase the production of dopamine, L-dopa and norepinephrine by 40%. This translates into improved sex drive, strength, vitality, mental clarity, alertness, overall energy production and a deceleration of age-related cognitive decline.

NADA and Immunity

While Enada is a key factor in the proper function of the Krebs Cycle, it is also responsible for initiating what is known as the "metabolic burst" This occurs during the immune response when a foreign invader attacks the body To mount an attack, this metabolic activity of macrophages, a specialized white blood cell that engulfs and destroys harmful substances, accelerates. The killing mechanism associated with this process, known as phagocytosis, is fueled by NADA.

Additional Benefits of NADA

- Acts as a free radical scavenger.
- Repairs DNA materials.
- Increases cellular energy.
- Protects liver from alcohol damage.
- Lowers cholesterol and decreases appetite.
- Assists in energizing the mitochondria.
- Used in the treatment of Parkinson's and Alzheimer's disease.
- Used to treat Chronic Fatigue Syndrome.

Dosage and Toxicity

Due to its safety of use, Enada's dose range can be customized to individual health and/or training needs. According to results of clinical trials by Dr. Birkmayer, I strongly suggest that you initially follow the manufacture's guidelines. NADA works best when taken on an empty stomach, 20-30 minutes before a meal, preferably in the morning. It is usually sold in 5mg (milligrams) tablets or capsules.

Food Sources

NADA is found in appreciable amounts in a variety of foods.

Pyruvate

Pyruvate is a relatively new product to the marketplace. It is, however, causing quite a stir. Chemically, pyruvate is composed of carbon, hydrogen and oxygen making it a carbohydrate. Pyruvate occurs naturally in the body and is involved with the metabolism of sugar and starches. It assists in the transportation of glucose into muscle cells. Studied extensively by Dr. Ronald Stanko, M.D., of the Gastroenterologic and Clinical Nutrition Division of the University of Pittsburgh Medical Center, pyruvate was investigated for its ability to naturally burn body fat. In fact, research by Dr. Stanko and co-workers have revealed that when pyruvate was administered to obese women for three weeks, they lost 37% more weight (13 vs. 9.5lbs) and 48% more fat 8.8 vs. 5.9 lbs.) than a control group. Additional studies have shown that pyruvate can also be effective without extensive exercise routines.

Pyruvate and Endurance

During the course of Dr. Stanko's investigations, an added benefit of pyruvate's use was discovered. Pyruvate increased muscle endurance by 20%, thus enabling athletes to increase the duration of their workouts with less perceived physical exertion, meaning physical tasks were much easier to complete due to increased energy. The reason for pyruvate's ability to increase endurance, stamina and exercise performance is directly related to its ability to facilitate the transport of glucose (blood sugar) into the muscle cell. This is known as "glucose extraction" and is concerned with how efficiently glucose from circulating blood is "utilized" by the muscle.

To put this extraction process into perspective, think of the last time you had a tune-up done on your car and the increase in its power after the tune-up was done. If you are able to somehow increase the efficiency at which your body extracts and then utilizes glucose (your high-test fuel), you could, effectively tune up your system. This is what pyruvate does.

Additionally, pyruvate is present in all human cells and is responsible for the release of the energy molecule "ATP".

The most important thing to remember is that pyruvate is not an artificial booster like coffee, caffeine or other stimulants.

Additional Benefits of Pyruvate

Regular oral dosages can reduce oxygen demands by the heart. Also, pyruvate:

- Has antioxidant capabilities.
- Stimulates metabolism.
- Improves cardiac function.
- Can reduce fat and unwanted cholesterol deposits.
- Can stimulate cellular mitochondrial respiration thus increasing the amount of energy for use by the mitochondria.

Suggested dose range is 5 grams a day, divided into 3 equal dosages, with meals. No serious side affects have been found with pyruvate.

Food Sources

Pyruvate is found in such foods as apples, cheeses, red wines, and a variety of other types of food, but only in minimal amounts.

Conclusion

Based on current thinking, due to a host of environmental, metabolic, aged-related, food-processing, soil variability and immune related disorders, non-essential accessory supplementation is a must. As cited in reports from the NIH (National Institute of Health), closing the gap of present day nutritional inadequacies via supplementation makes good sense.

While this book cannot cover the entire array of accessory energizing supplements, their use, however, has skyrocketed. Many people experience noticeable increases in their energy levels when they also take supplements from the following list.

- Bee Pollen
- Glycerol
- Cordyceps Sinesis
- Essential Fatty Acids
- Evening Primrose Oil
- Glandular Extracts
- Inosine
- Lecithin
- Malic Acid
- Medium Chain Triglycerides (MCT Fuels)
- Octacosonal
- Peppermint
- Phospatidyl Serine
- Super Oxide Dismutase (SOD)

The most exciting things about these accessory supplements are that many of them strengthen or are part of the natural metabolic cycle that produces energy. Also many of these supplements compliment or enhance the workings of internal organs as well as encourage strong immune responses.

Amino Acids

"Protein also contributes to the body's overall energy metabolism. After removal of the nitrogenous portion of the amino acid, the remaining part may be converted to fat or carbohydrate. If there is not sufficient carbohydrate or fat available in the diet for energy, then as much as 58% of the total dietary protein found in the amino acid pool is utilized for energy."

Dr. Sue Rodwell Williams. Ph.D., R.D.
Chief, Nutrition Program
Kaiser-Permanent Medical Center, 1978

One of the most researched areas today is the issue of how we age and why metabolic systems wear out. For years, scientists have tried to unlock the secret of the "biological clock" ticking inside you. If we could somehow rejuvenate, repair, and/or rebuild our organ systems, we could maintain stability and create an internal environment for the creation and proper utilization of energy. This is, in essence, the role of amino acids, known as the "building blocks of life".

Amino acids are the metabolic end result of the protein that has been extracted and broken down from the food you eat. Proteins, like those from steak, nuts, and cheese, are too large to pass into the bloodstream. Once broken down, protein is transformed into smaller pieces called amino acids. These dynamic substances are responsible for re-building our bodies. Our cells, hair, teeth, fingernails, blood, arteries, veins, hormones and organs are all made from protein.

Simply put, we are "protein beings". Without an ample supply, we are susceptible to an array of negative health disorders. For example, one of the major causes of fatigue is inadequate protein intake. Proteins are involved in the composition of cells and muscular contractions. In fact, next to water, protein is the most essential constituent of cellular metabolic components. In other words, proteins and amino acids are the materials from which our internal energy mechanism is made.

The Amino Acid Pool

How important is it that you maintain proper levels of amino acids? Very important. In fact, if you don't, your body will rob existing muscle tissue to provide the bloodstream with the correct proportions of the amino acids it needs. This phenomenon is known as catabolism. The body seeks to maintain what scientists call its "free amino acid pool". To do this, nutritionists suggest that we eat 4 or 5 small meals a day as opposed to two large ones. This practice helps to maintain more stable blood sugar and energy levels and prevents or slows down the catabolic process, thus encouraging building of body tissue and structures.

Non-Essential and Essential Amino Acids

Presently there are twenty-two known amino acids. Fourteen of these amino acids are considered to be non-essential, meaning that under ideal situations and in the absence of any metabolic disorders, the body is capable of producing its own supply. They are:

- Aspartic Acid
- Carnitine
- Citrulline
- Cysteine
- Cystine
- Gamma-Aminobutuyric Acid (GABA)
- Glutamic Acid
- Glycine
- Histidine
- Norleucine
- Ornithine
- Proline
- Serine
- Tyrosine

The essential amino acids, those that absolutely must be supplied through your diet because the body is incapable of making them, are:

- Isoleucine
- Leucine
- Lysine
- Methionine
- Phenylalanine
- Threonine
- Tryptophan
- Valine

Many researchers consider this division of amino acids to be a misnomer (incorrect label) because, from a biological and metabolic standpoint, all twenty-two are needed in the proper portions at the same time to maintain optimum health.

While all the amino acids are important, we shall review a few that are very popular due to their ability to enhance natural metabolic activity.

Special Note: *Amino acids are designed by either "L" (such as L-Lysine) or by a "D" (such as DL Phenylalanine). L-Forms are in their natural state. They are biologically active, in the L-Form (ready for use by human tissue). D-Forms are in a synthetic or artificial state. Look for the "L" designation when purchasing them.*

Special Note: "L" and "D" refer to the rotation of light by the molecules. Nature's preferences are not arbitrary since the "L" form hooks up properly in metabolic partnering.

The Amino Acids

A. Branch Chain Amino Acids

Before we take a look at the individual metabolic attributes of a few of the amino acids, I would first like to introduce a special group of amino acids. They are known as the "Branch Chain Aminos". They are named as such due to their molecular configuration. The branch chain aminos are: isoleucine, leucine, and valine. What is important about these three aminos is the fact that they make up about 1/3 of all of the protein found in your muscles.

While we have looked, throughout this book, at energy and how it is generated, let's intensify our focus and talk a little about what actually causes fatigue to set in. First of all, every move you make is powered by glycogen that is made and stored for use by your body. However, whenever you do physical work — walking, exercising, gardening, jogging, swimming etc. — the body produces a by-product called "lactic acid". Muscles do not function well in a lactic acid environment, and fatigue sets in.

When you exercise regularly lactic acid build-up and muscular fatigue is less prevalent. Exercising keeps the pump of your circulatory system primed, so that it will remove lactic acid much quicker, thus resulting in less fatigue.

There is, however, another built-in system the body uses to minimize this muscular fatigue. This back-up system, as I'm sure you have guessed, is via the use of the branch chain amino acids present in muscle tissue. The body uses the branch chain amino acids as an indirect energy supply for muscles, by connecting them to glucose by a process known as "gluconeogenesis". The process of gluconeogenesis is very prevalent in individuals who restrict their calorie intake or go on semi-starvation diets.

B. Branch Chains and Central Fatigue

While all amino acids will supply needed fuel under some extenuating circumstances, researchers have confirmed that branch chain amino acids can be utilized much more effectively. As cited by J. Mark Davis of the Department of Exercise Science, at the University of South Carolina in Columbia, fatigue can also result from alterations within the "Central Nervous System" (CNS). Studies have shown that especially after a strenuous workout the central nervous system recovery can take days, leaving you psychologically drained. This can have a negative impact in your attempts to continue and/or muster up the energy necessary to proceed with your scheduled workout routines.

In fact, according to Mr. Davis, the lack of central nervous system drive to the working muscles is the most likely explanation of fatigue in most people during normal activities. New research and trials conducted with certain amino acids such as GABA, tyrosine, phenylalanine and the branch chain amino acids imply that all possibly delay central fatigue. This is due, in part, to the fact that they are, as cited by Dr. J.D. Fernstrom, Ph.D., (Professor of Psychiatry, Pharmacology and Behavioral Neuro-Science at the University of Pittsburgh School of Medicine), precursors of several central nervous system neurotransmitters.

By increasing the concentrations of branch chain aminos in the bloodstream, one can possibly "trick" the body into producing less concentrations of trytophan. This amino acid has been implicated as a possible factor in accelerating "CNS" fatigue during prolonged exercise.

Studies suggest that by ingesting certain foods which are abundant in these amino acids or the drinking of carbohydrate rich drinks which includes BCAA's you will go a long way in shifting your energy levels from neutral to turbo-drive!

Additional Benefits of Branch Chain Amino Acids

- Help prevent muscle protein wasting or breakdown
- Spare stored muscle glycogen
- Assist in releasing of growth hormone

Dosage and Toxicity

When using Branch Chain Amino Acids please follow suggested dosage guidelines. Reported studies have shown that 7-12 grams taken during exercise will slow down protein breakdown. This will help preserve one of your most powerful metabolic agents, namely your own muscle tissue.

Food Sources

Excellent food sources of branch chain amino acids are whey protein, meats and dairy products. Whey protein can be purchased in vitamin and health food stores.

Carnitine

Carnitine's use was popularized by individuals engaged in weight training to build muscle. They used carnitine because its main function is that of fat burning. Today carnitine is used by athletes, joggers, cyclists, marathon runners, and those individuals looking to shed unwanted pounds. The specific action of carnitine is that of breaking down fats into fatty acids. Like coal being shoveled into a furnace, fatty acids are transported into the cell's mitochondria to be burned as fuel.

This action is similar to the process in which the carburetor in your car controls the flow of gasoline into its engine. As this fuel burns, it supplies the impetus to move your car. Similarly, carnitine frees stored body fat from fat cells in a process called lipolysis, to be used as a fuel. An added plus here is a reduction in body fat, which contributes to a more sleek and slender you.

Additional Benefits of Carnitine

- Preserves muscle glycogen (fuel) during exercise
- Encourages the disposal of triglycerides (body fats)
- Prevents the buildup of deadly ketones (by-products of insufficient carbohydrate metabolism)
- May improve various neuromuscular diseases
- Can improve heart function and tolerance

Special Note: *Protein amino acids are not the body's preferred source of fuel. However, when fats and carbohydrates are in short supply, as during illness, intense training, exercise, and in certain dieting situations, the body will burn Branch Chain Amino Acids, which are, as previously discussed, metabolized directly in muscle tissue. It is carnitine that facilitates this process.*

Dosage and Toxicity

In clinical trials, dose ranges of 1 to 15 grams presented no side-effects, except short-term diarrhea. Suggested dosage, 500mg (milligrams) daily.

Food Sources

Found in protein-containing foods such as meat, fish, and chicken.

Tyrosine

This non-essential amino acid has gained much attention for its ability to fight depression by naturally modulating the affects of neurotransmitters. As a point of reference, neurotransmitters help control the flow of signals from the brain to other parts of the body. The reason for such interest in Tyrosine is in part due to its production of norepinephrine, epinephrine and dopamine. All of these brain chemicals are excitatory in nature. They are responsible for elevating mood, thus stimulating alertness, energy and an overall feeling of exhilaration.

Closely related to the amino acid Phenylalanine in its actions, scientists sometimes regard these as one in the same. Tyrosine naturally blocks the absorption of tryptophan, the amino acid which is responsible for inducing sleep and relaxed states. Tyrosine would be most beneficial to the heavy caffeine and coffee drinker as a replacement pick-me-up prior to exercising.

In addition to the above, tyrosine is now being used as an adjunct treatment for cocaine addiction, and its withdrawal symptoms (extreme irritability and fatigue). Researchers also claim that by supplementing one to three grams of tyrosine 20-30 minutes before a high carbohydrate meal-such as pasta, spaghetti, or pizza, you may be able to avoid the sluggish feeling that usually follows.

Additional Benefits of Tyrosine

- Helps reduce stress and anxiety
- Can help suppress appetite
- Stimulates growth hormone release and muscular growth
- May inhibit age-related loss of hair pigment
- Has antioxidant capabilities, scavenging free radicals

Dosage and Toxicity

Suggested dosage is 100 mg (milligrams) or lower. Tyrosine should not be used with prescription "MAO" inhibitors. MAO inhibitors include certain antidepressant drugs. Individuals with blood pressure abnormalities should use caution. Tyrosine has a tendency to lower blood pressure rather than increase it.

Food Sources

Chicken, fish, eggs, animal and plant protein sources.

Glutamine

This amino acid has recently been the subject of numerous scientific studies. As the most abundant amino acid in skeleton tissue (61%) it is known for its ability to accelerate protein synthesis, as well as muscle, immune, and gastrointestinal function. Glutamine, as a protein synthesizer, is used in hospitals to offset the trauma and muscle wasting burn victims often experience.

In addition to the above, Glutamine is a powerful brain energy booster. Glutamine actually buffers or removes ammonia from the brain area. Ammonia can inhibit the proper firing of brain neurotransmitters. In the buffering process, it also helps alleviate depression and the fatigue associated with it as well as stimulating natural growth hormone release. Growth hormone is secreted by the pituitary gland in the brain and is responsible for growth and repair, plus stimulating immune function. Furthermore, glutamine helps maintain cellular hydration or cell volume.

Cell Volumizing

Cell volumizing is a new concept that refers to a natural "shuttle service" of nutrients into the cell, especially water and protein. Scientists contend that during this process, the body actually signals the muscles to utilize protein more productively for building and glycogen (stored fuel in the muscles) use. Glutamine, with the aid of the amino acid glycine, work together in facilitating this natural process. Additionally, glutamine (not carbohydrates or fats) is the fuel source preferred by cells that divide at a rapid pace called entercytes (intestinal cells) and lymphocytes. Lymphocytes are a type of white blood cells that defend against foreign invaders into the system.

Glutamine and Your Energy Blueprint

Aside from the benefits listed above, glutamine is actively involved with a number of different metabolic pathways. Dr. Brian Liebovitz, Ph.D., a well-known nutritional biochemist states:

"The extent of glutamine's involvement in the complex metabolism of the human body is awesome."

Dr. Liebovitz also maintains that Sir Hans Krebs, the scientist who first suggested the existence of our metabolic pathways, made the following statements concerning glutamine's enormous role in precipitating metabolic actions:

Apart from being a protein and peptide constituent, it plays a role in the acid-base balance as a precursor of ordinary ammonia. It is a precursor (before the next step in the formation of) amino sugars, and plays a role in detoxification. It is a nitrogen carrier, it is a regulator of hepatic (pertaining to the liver) glycogen synthesis and it is a reparatory fuel in certain tissues.

Dr. Liebovitz goes on to say that "while most amino acids have multiple functions, glutamine however appears to be the most versatile."

Additional Benefits of Glutamine

- Assists in the disposal of uric acid (toxic by-product of protein metabolism)
- Improves memory, attention and alertness
- Can help support brain fuel needs in the absence of glucose (the brain's major fuel source)
- Can reduce severity of associated negative affects of chemotherapy

Dosage and Toxicity

Suggested dose range 1000 to 4000 mg a day in divided dosages.

Food Sources

Found primarily in animal and plant sources. Raw spinach and parsley are excellent sources.

Please Note: Glutamine is destroyed very rapidly by heat when foods are cooked. I highly recommend supplementation to augment food-based sources.

Other Important Amino Acids

Glycine: This amino acid is an active participant in muscle cell metabolism. It is naturally converted into creatine, which acts as the high energy agent supplying energy for muscle contractions.

Taurine: Strengthens normal brain wave patterns for mental clarity and alertness.

GABA: Stimulates neurotransmitter activity and functions as an anti-stress, anti-anxiety, and general relaxing agent.

Tryptophan: This amino acid will help you relax and can aid you as a natural sleep aid. Found abundantly in milk, hence the reason some people drink warm or hot milk before going to sleep.

Note: *You can only purchase tryptophan as part of a naturally occurring amino acid complex. You can, however, purchase its precursor called*

5-Hydroxtryptophan (5-HTP) which in clinical trials have been shown to be equally as effective. Tryptophan supplements were removed from the market place several years ago due to an outbreak of eosinophilia (a rare blood disorder) now known to have been caused by contamination by a Japanese firm's raw materials and not by tryptophan itself.

Enzymes

"Various names such as life energy, life force, life principle, vitality, vital force, strength, and nerve energy have been offered to describe this energy. Without the life energy of enzymes we would be nothing more than a pile of lifeless chemical substances. Both maintaining health and in healing, enzymes and only enzymes do the actual work. They are what we call in metabolism, the body's labor force."

Dr. Edward Howell
Enzyme Nutrition — The Food Concept

As we learned in Chapter One, many of the chemical reactions in nature, without enzymes, would occur at such slow rates they wouldn't be done fast enough to satisfy human metabolic needs. When you think about the enormous power enzymes have, you are able to understand why they are referred to as the "life force". Enzymes are defined as biological catalysts that initiate and accelerate chemical reactions, without being changed themselves in the process.

New Thinking on Enzymes

Scientists once believed that the body has an unlimited amount of enzymes. Researchers now know that the body's supply and power of enzymes can diminish due to a number of factors. Based on research from leading universities, such as the University of Toronto, The Rockefeller Institute of Medicine, and Johns Hopkin University, new views have emerged regarding our enzyme potential. The following synopsis represents current knowledge about the nature of enzymes and their production:

1. The number of enzymes we are capable of making during our life span is not unlimited. We are born with an enzyme potential and that potential cannot be exceeded.
2. Enzymes are tireless workers. They are, however, exhaustible. When this happens they must somehow be replaced or replenished.
3. To a large degree, your life span, energy, and vitality is a reflection of how well your body can generate enough enzyme activity to keep your internal energy blueprint or metabolic pathway operating.

This new thinking concerning the efficacy of enzymes also has clearly established why we need to incorporate exogenous (outside) enzymes in our diet. In this way, the enzyme potential of those secreted naturally by the body will not have to be wasted to digest food. Much of their catalytic ability can then be shifted toward bio-energetic pathways and energy metabolism.

The Types of Enzymes

Enzymes are classified as either metabolic, digestive, or food enzymes. Metabolic enzymes run your body, while digestive enzymes digest your food, and food enzymes start the digestion process.

At this point I am sure you can visualize the overall importance of these substances, in terms of your energy potential. If enzymes actually run your body and help breakdown your food so that it is small enough to enter the bloodstream, your internal metabolic processes will be incapable of functioning properly without them.

Additionally, as stated above, food enzymes start the digestive process. Research has confirmed that enzymes naturally present in foods, are destroyed when food is cooked. Heat destroys enzymes very rapidly. Due to the highly processed nature of many foods, health officials now claim that we are essentially eating "enzyme-less" food. This puts an enormous burden on the body to make the necessary enzymes. The burden is complicated by the fact that no one enzyme has the ability to digest all types of foods and most enzymes are, in fact, quite specific in their functions. There are literally hundreds of combinations used to digest certain types of foods.

Table 5.1 Digestive Enzymes

Digestive Fluid	Enzyme	Substance Acted Upon	Products Formed
Saliva	Salivary amylase	Boiled starch and dextrins	Dextrin and maltose
Gastric Juices	Pepsin	Protein	Polypeptides and clotted milk
	Gastric lipase	Emulsified fat	Fatty acids and glycerol
Pancreatic Juice	Tyrosine	Proteins Chymotrypsinogen	Polypeptides Chymotrypsin
	Chymotrypsin	Proteins	Polypeptides
	Carboxypolypeptidase	Polypeptides	Peptides & amino acids
	Pancreatic amylase	Starch and dextrin's	Maltose
	Pancreatic lipase	fat	Fatty acids, and glycerol

Table 5.1 — Courtesy of: King and Showers, *Human Anatomy and Physiology*; W.B. Sauders, Philadelphia, PA; 1969, 6th ed.; pg.361

In considering the initiating and controlling capabilities of these powerful substances, consider the words of Dr. Ivan Kelly, an enzyme researcher:

As living things, our general health depends directly on the specific health of our enzymes. If they are youthful and vigorous, we will exhibit radiant energy. But if they are weak, and worn, we become candidates for general malaise (a condition of body weakness) and premature aging.

In addition to those enzymes listed in table 5.1, other plant-based enzymes such as bromelain (found in pineapples), papain (commonly known as papaya) and apple pectin (from apples) are excellent sources of digestive enzymes.

Herbs

"We know well that the herb can and does assimilate inorganic (non-living) mineral matter, and through some mysterious and unknown way convert this inert (no ability to react) and lifeless matter into living organic material, which when presented to the animal or human cell, is hungrily absorbed, sustaining and renewing its life's process."

Dr. Edward E. Shook
Advanced Treatise in Herbology

Herbs are one of the oldest categories of products possessing medicinal value. Built around early folklore and anecdotal (word of mouth) evidence, herbs have gained popularity and are now firmly grounded in scientific evidence concerning their safety and effectiveness. While many cultures have traditionally used herbal preparations to treat a wide range of both physical and mental problems, they are, however, just beginning to gain acceptance by the medical community here in the U.S. for their health-promoting capabilities.

This is perplexing since, according to the World Health Organization, nearly 80 percent of the planet's population relies on traditional medicine, namely herbal remedies, as a primary source of health care. Also a significant number of biomedical drugs on the market come directly from the plant kingdom. Approximately 25% of all prescription drugs used in the United States today contain compounds based on prototype parent molecules originally isolated from plants. Out of 120 drugs of natural product origin on the market today, 74% were discovered based on their history of use as traditional medicines. These 120 drugs come from only 90 out of an estimated 250,000 known angiosperms (flowering plants). These figures underscore the therapeutic value and potential of numerous medicinal plants.

Dr. Earl Mindell, one of the nation's foremost health, botanical and pharmacological experts, agrees with the above findings. In fact, he maintains that prior to World War II, herbal medications were listed side-by-side with chemical drugs in the US Pharmacopoeia, the official listing of accepted medicines. Additionally, he claims that nearly 50% of the thousands of drugs commonly used and prescribed are either derived from a plant source or contain chemical substances of a plant compound. The following synopsis outlines a few common drugs you may be aware of:

- Digitalis — a potent cardiotonic, it is derived from the Fox Glove plant.
- Aspirin — a chemical imitation of salicin from the bark of the white willow tree.
- Reserpine — a blood pressure medication, it is actually an ancient Indian remedy derived from an Asian shrub.
- Ephedrine and pseudoephedrine — found in many over-the-counter cold remedies, these are derived from the ephedra plant, which has been used in China to treat colds and flu for more than 5,000 years.
- Penicillin — the grandfather of antibiotics, it is actually a mold, an organism produced by a fungus, a primitive plant.

What Is An Herb?

An herb is defined as a flowering plant whose above ground stem does not become woody, which is valued for its medicinal properties. Herbs have the capability to trap the energy of sunlight. Herbs are intimately involved with the human bioenergetic process. Herbs, are pharmacologically *alive*. They can and do exert positive effects on human energetics.

When plants and herbs are metabolized, they are actually releasing the enormous power of nature. Therefore, in their constituent form, herbs have the ability to augment natural metabolic pathways.

Herbs Are Synergistic

One of the most important and attractive aspects of herbs compared to drugs is the fact that herbs are "synergistic". Synergism refers to the ability of a group of substances to have a stronger effect than a single substances alone. For example, the combination of Siberian ginseng, gotu kola, bee pollen and cayenne, may have a more profound impact on depression and boosting energy levels than any of the herbs individually.

Studies have confirmed that herbs are synergistic and perform better when used in this manner. An added benefit here is the safety involved in doing this. As is the case with most things in nature, herbs are not packaged as isolated chemicals. The active constituents in herbs come with substances which help offset possible negative effects. For instance, ephedrine, which comes from the ma huang plant can cause high blood pressure in some sensitive individuals. However, when the whole plant is used, data indicates that the negative aspects are diminished.

How are Herbs Used?

Herbal preparations can be purchased without a doctor's prescription. However, herbs should be viewed as mild medicines having the ability in some cases to accelerate the actions of certain prescription drugs. For this reason, it is not advisable to cultivate your own herbs without professional guidelines as many plant species have potentially toxic capabilities.

Herbs generally used for medicinal purposes are found in liquid tinctures and extracts as well as powders, capsules, teas, and/or tablets for internal consumption.

The Standardized Revolution

Over the last several years, in an effort to insure that the active ingredients are intact after processing an herb, researchers have begun to standardize them. One of the major problems with herbs is their variability. The constituents that affect their elemental properties — sunlight, temperature and soil quality, as well as processing and storage procedures — all affect the herb's potency. When an herb is standardized, certain levels or percentages of its active ingredient is present in the finished product.

In the past, all herbal preparations were identified as a plant/extract ratio, ranging in potencies from 4:1 to 500:1. In this example, an herbal product being 100mg at a 4-1 (4:1) concentration was produced from 400 mg (milligrams) of the herb, but actually only yields 100 mg of extracted powder or liquid. The problem here is, of the 100 mg product that is left, what percentage of the active ingredients can be found in it. The goal of standardization is to insure that the herb's effectiveness is not compromised. By insuring that a certain percentage of the active constituents are present, you are assured of getting some genuine portion of the herb instead of possible non-active, inert material.

Cayenne (Capsicum)

Cayenne (Capsicumfrutoscens) is a group of herbal plants that are part of the pepper family. This family includes red jalapeno and bell peppers, mild paprika and actually all other herbs. Cayenne is best known for its ability to increase circulation, thus stimulating the entire body because of its ability to cause the natural release of endorphins in the brain. Endorphins are brain chemicals that help us resist pain and naturally maintain feelings of euphoria, exhilaration, and cheerfulness.

Cayenne also has an extraordinary effect on metabolism, enhancing the body's ability to burn up calories, and aiding it in digestion. It also accelerates glucose metabolism, providing the body and brain with this much needed fuel.

Additional Benefits of Cayenne

- Excellent stimulant for sluggishness
- Has powerful antioxidant capabilities
- Can be used to treat arthritic disturbances
- Relieves gastric discomfort

When combined with the herb lobelia, cayenne is excellent as a nervine (calming agent).

Ginseng

Ginseng is one of the most well-known herbal supplements used in the United States. The use and application of this herb was first recorded in the "Shen Nung Pen Yasho Ching". This work, a pharmacopoeia (book containing a list of drugs, their formulas usages and other related information), is cited as being written in the second century B.C.

Ginseng's ability to increase energy, especially at the cellular level, is due to its activity as an "adaptogen". Adaptogens are substances that help you handle various stresses. The latest research on adaptogenic substances reveal that they help the cells to build "energy factories" by activating certain "workers", including MRNA (messenger) and +RNA (transportation). RNA, which stands for ribonucleic acid, is responsible for translating the genetic message from the DNA molecule. Deoxyribonucleic Acid is responsible for making protein from amino acids. DNA is said to contain the blueprint for human construction, while RNA makes sure its commands and messages are carried out properly.

The Anatomy of an Adaptogen

As previously stated, adaptogens are substances that have the ability to increase metabolic actions, to build resistance, and to strengthen the entire body. To fall under this classification, adaptogens should:

1. Be non-toxic, creating a minimal amount of disruption to normal metabolic functions.
2. Be target originated, having the ability to increase resistance against an array of negative factors that may be physical, chemical or biological in nature.
3. Have the ability to stabilize or move bodily functions toward homeostasis, regardless of direction or movement toward an unhealthy state.

The principles outlined by the renowned physiologist I. I. Beckman, gave classification to adaptogens, and their ability to bring bodily functions into balance. For example, if blood sugar levels are low or if blood pressure is too high, an adaptogen (like ginseng) will help bring them back to normal levels, states Dr. Earl Mindell, whom I spoke of earlier. According to Dr. Mindell, ginseng acts on the pituitary gland helping to regulate blood sugar and support adrenal function, generally promoting physical and mental alertness and creating energy and stamina.

In essence, ginseng has the ability to normalize body functions by assisting it in utilizing substances, while helping to eliminate harmful toxic materials.

The Many Faces of Ginseng

There are many different kinds of ginseng, all with varying properties. American ginseng, known as (panax quinquefolium) is a classic adaptogen. Korean ginseng, best known as panax ginseng, is highly stimulating. It is most suited for immediate energy needs. It can be purchased in either red or white forms with both having similar properties.

Note: *Red is cured and is considered to be more Yang (more immediate energy). White is more Yin (or balanced) since ginseng is considered quite Yang to begin with.*

Siberian ginseng, "Eleutherococcus Senticosus", comes from Siberia and is not botanically related to American or Korean Ginseng. Siberian ginseng became popular when the Russian Olympic team used it as a dietary adjunct to support physical energy needs during training. In experiments with animals, the Russians had discovered that work capacity could be increased by 25 to 70 percent depending on the dose administered. Siberian ginseng is also classified as an adaptogen.

As a point of reference, adaptogens usually exhibit long term effects at building energy and are not particularly useful for immediate energy needs.

Pharmacological Properties

The medicinal value of ginseng is attributed to substances known as "ginsenosides" or "saponins". These substances are naturally occurring compounds and have a profound effect on human bioenergies. Studies have shown that these saponins or ginsenosides (found in American and Korean ginseng) can:

- Have a tranquilizing effect to the central nervous system and acts as an anti-fatigue agent.
- Act on proteins in the liver and bone marrow cells, thus building immunity.

The active components, which share some similar functions in Siberian ginseng, are called "eleutherocides". Studies have revealed that eleutherocides may have a slight advantage over the ginsenosides in panax ginseng (Korean and American). Researchers have found that Siberian ginseng's energy-producing effects lasted longer and were more profound in an intense physical work setting. Additionally, Siberian ginseng showed the ability to have a more calming or normalizing effect than that of a stimulant such as panax ginseng.

This may make eleutherococcus senticosus (Siberian ginseng) more attractive to those of you who are pre-disposed toward high blood pressure and or high anxiety. *Please check with your health care professional if you fall into this category before you take ginseng.*

Additional Benefits of Ginseng

- Assists in coronary circulation and normalizing arterial pressures
- Stimulates protein and lipid (fat) metabolism
- Helps stabilize blood glucose levels
- Has antioxidant capabilities, reducing oxidation and the formation of free radicals
- Inhibits abnormal cell growth and assists spleen and lymphatic functions, thus enhancing resistance to disease
- Helps control blood pressure
- Stimulates the metabolic functions of the liver, kidney and other organs
- Can help raise low blood pressure
- Can induce sweating, thus serving as a detoxifier
- Stimulates appetite and can be used to help normalize digestive disorders.
- Has possible aphrodisiac capabilities

Dosage and Toxicity

There is no recommended dosage for ginseng. Some studies suggest 100 to 200 mg of standardized extracts (4 to 7% ginsenosides) of panax ginseng per day. For siberian ginseng, 300 to 400 mg a day. You will probably have to find your optimal level through trial and error. However, I strongly advise that you follow established manufacturer guidelines on usage. Also, if you have high blood pressure, you should consult your health care professional before usage. This herb should not be used by pregnant or lactating women.

Dong Quai
(Angelica Sinensis)

One of the most famous botanicals in China, Dong Quai is prized for it's ability to help alleviate a number of gynecological problems. Because of this fact, it is known as the "Female Ginseng". Dong Quai can fortify the female reproductive system, diminish the effects of hot flashes, and help regulate PMS (pre-menstrual symptoms).

Herbalists contend that this herb, rich in many nutrients, may help prevent anemia in both men and women and can rejuvenate the blood.

Licorice
(Glycyrrihiza glaba)

While many people enjoy the taste of licorice, this herb is gaining popularity for its wide range of medicinal properties. Recent scientific studies have confirmed that the saponin found in licorice aids the secretion of several hormones. One hormone, aldosterone, decreases the kidney output of salt and water. The amount of salt and water in the body determines the volume of blood and interstitial fluids in the body. Aldosterone functions to build blood volume that keeps arterial (blood) pressure normal.

This action is important because continued stress, both physical and mental, can rapidly exhaust adrenal function and adversely effect your energy levels. The adrenal glands, one located above each of the kidneys, also secrete two other hormones, epinephrine and nonepinephrine. Both of these hormones influence metabolism and act on the central nervous system.

Epinephrine and Norepinephrine

Epinephrine is a potent stimulative hormone that has powerful hyperglycemic actions, increasing blood sugar levels (your circulating energy). Licorice stimulates the production of epinephrine thereby facilitating glycogenolysis (the conversion of carbohydrates stored in the liver and muscle into glucose). Epinephrine also accelerates the removal of free fatty acids from adipose (fat) tissues. When fat is broken down into fatty acids, these serve as an extremely powerful source of fuel, energizing the entire body.

Nonepinephrine, like epinephrine, has both stimulatory and inhibitory affects. Studies have shown it to have a less powerful stimulative effect than its counterpart, epinephrine. It is also, however, involved with carbohydrate metabolism (your main fuel source) and the liberation of fat for use as a energy source. Epinephrine also helps provide the energy needed in stressful or "physically" dangerous situations. This hormone is found to be secreted more in species that are highly aggressive.

Because of the above factors, deglycyrrhizanted licorice is considered to be one of the most effective adaptogens that enhances normal adrenal functions.

Additional Benefits of Licorice

- Encourages sound immune responses
- Serves as an excellent expectorant
- Beneficial for sore throats
- Excellent as a cough suppressant
- Increases secretions of gastric juices from gastric mucosa, thus helping to heal ulcers.

Dosage and Toxicity

Suggested dose range from 200 to 600 mg. Make sure your extract or tablet has been standardized for "glycyrrhizin" content. Do not use licorice if you have high blood pressure. The glycyrrhizin alkaloids do not contain as many of the compounds found in standard licorice that raise blood pressure.

The herbalist Christopher Hobbs recommends simmering three to five grams of licorice in two and one half (2½) cups of water for 30 minutes. Consume half in the morning and the other half in the evening to fortify the adrenals.

St. John's Wort
(Hypericum Perforatum)

St. John's Wort is very popular in Germany where it is used as an approved treatment for depression. In fact, in 1993 some 217 million prescriptions a year were written by physicians in Germany for hypericum. This is twenty-five times the amount of prescriptions that were written for the popular anti-depressant drug Prozac here in the United States.

The major reason for this herb's popularity is that its side effects are less serious than that of traditional anti-depressants. Anti-depressants drugs can cause weight loss, insomnia and in some cases sexual dysfunction. In clinical trials, however, St. John's Wort only exhibited mild allergic reactions and gastrointestinal irritations in limited instances. Additionally, anti-depressant drugs directly affect the chemistry of the brain and its processing.

Mood and Energy

St. John's Wort can serve as a natural mood elevator, an overall mental stimulator, and a nervous system tonic. An added benefit of the application of this medicinal herb is its ability to improve REM sleep. REM sleep is the deepest and most complete pattern of sleep. Research has shown that disorders in this sleep pattern can wreak havoc on energy levels, concentration, immune system function, and overall patterns of well-being.

Additional Benefits of Hypericum

- Acts as a muscle relaxer
- Used to treat menstrual cramps
- Serves as an expectorant
- May inhibit the growth of retro viruses
- Promotes healing of skin wounds

Dosage and Toxicity

Current data suggest that 300 milligrams of St. John's Wort, which has been standardized with at least 3% of its active component hypericum, three times a day is most effective. Although no toxicity problems have been associated with this herb, hypericum contains a photosensitizing substance and reacts with light. For this reason, light-skinned individuals should avoid sun-light when taking this herb.

Note: *St. John's Wort should not be used in conjunction with other anti-depressant drugs.*

Conclusions

Based on past and current data, herbal preparations have a long and safe history of use, dating as far back as 3,000 to 4,000 years B.C. While herbal remedies continue to be the major source of many of the drugs used today, they still are the primary remedies used in many parts of the world, in their unadulterated form. Nevertheless, there is still much skepticism concerning their efficacy here in the U.S.

This, however, is rapidly changing as Americans seek more non-invasive means to facilitate normal metabolic processes. Although herbs offer a wide range of benefits, they should be used judiciously, since they often contain minute amounts of the active alkaloids used to manufacture many of today's prescription drugs.

While there are many more herbs touted for their ability to stimulate or enhance human energy systems, modern medicine is just beginning to understand the nature of many new herbs. How medicinal plants are metabolized, including the order and specific values inside their cells and how these attributes are effectively transferred into cells of human physiology, remains a largely uncharted frontier. Herbs, however, truly are nature's prescription medicines!

In today's market, researchers claim that you can't rely on the proposed attributes of an herb if the percentage of active components used aren't listed on the label with corresponding percentages. Because of the above factors, look for herbs that have been standardized or from a supplier of known quality.

Note: *It is worth mentioning that a new generation of broad or "full spectrum" standardized herbal products are entering the marketplace which are standardized on a range of active constituents. These are the* *results of a realization that the synergistic qualities of the herbs are based on more than one active constituent. They also prevent "spiking" of inert material with a single standardized constituent.*

Vitamins and Minerals

"I was wrong about vitamins and minerals. Twenty years ago I told my television viewers that most people didn't need vitamins. I certainly wasn't alone in this belief. At the time, few people in the medical community supported supplementation. I now know that my previous pronouncements simply aren't true. No matter what your age, no matter what your health status, according to new research, optimum dosages of vitamins and minerals can improve your health."

Dr. Art Ulene
Physician, Author and
Television Personality

Vitamins and minerals are by far the most well-known of all supplements. While studies continue to show a steady increase in the number of Americans (about 50% of the population) who take vitamin and mineral supplements, their overall role is still misunderstood. This is evidenced by the opening remarks of Dr. Ulene, whose views, and others like his, took some twenty years to reverse. With the advances in the study of nutrition, scientists now contend that nutritional supplements are an important part of an overall health program. According to Jeffrey Blumberg of the USDA Human Nutrition Research Center on Aging at Tufts University, research during the past two decades now clearly indicates that vitamins and minerals play an important role in promoting optimal health and in preventing chronic diseases.

Based on mounting research, more and more scientists are starting to realize that traditional medical views on vitamins and minerals have been too limited. That sentiment was recently expressed by Dr. Lawrence Machlin, Director of Human Research at Hoffman-LaRoche, Inc. in a paper presented at the New York Academy of Sciences Symposium, entitled "Beyond Deficiency:

New Views on the Function and Health Effects of Vitamins and Minerals."

In light of these new findings many health officials advocate an individualized vitamin and supplement program for nearly everyone. In fact, according to Elizabeth Somer, M.A., R.D., a well-known and widely respected nutritionist, the latest research shows that eating well and taking supplements is not an either/or issue. For optimum health you need to do both.

- Just what are vitamins and minerals?
- How do they produce energy?
- What are antioxidants?
- What do they have to do with energy levels?
- How do vitamins and minerals work?

Like their enzyme counterparts, vitamins and minerals function as co-enzymes for many of your metabolic cycles. While enzymes start and initiate virtually every metabolic process in the body, they sometimes need a little help from a partner, co-factor or co-enzyme, which are the vitamins and minerals. Directly then, vitamins and minerals play a major role in how your body produces energy.

For example, many of the B-vitamins are responsible for turning the food you consume into fuel. Many of the minerals found in your body can be thought of as being the electrical spark plugs found in your car, or its battery. Car batteries run off of positive and negative electrical cables which supply the energy to start your car. Similarly ionized minerals carry particular charges which allow electrical currents to pass through them in the solution of your body. The following analogy will give you a simplified view of the co-partner nature of vitamins and minerals and their relationship to human energetics.

#1
Your car is essentially useless without a key and someone to turn it.
#2
Your car however has an ignition.

#3
When the right key is inserted and turned
#4
The engine is started and the car becomes a powerful entity.
#5

However, the engine started only because the car battery was charged and had no dead cells which might slow down or inhibit its starting power.

In this simple analogy your body represents the car and your car keys the biological enzymes that must be present to start or turn the engine over. The battery in your car corresponds to the vitamins and minerals, the co-factors or co-enzymes that must be present to supply power to other parts of your body or, in our analogy, of your car. When vitamins and minerals are not present in optimum amounts, your ability to reach or sustain your full energy potential is severely compromised. A full complement of these tiny, but powerful, supplements should be part of any general health-building or energy therapy program.

The Antioxidant Connection

Current data has conclusively shown that vitamins and minerals have powerful antioxidant capabilities. Antioxidants are considered to be one of the most important discoveries in the medical history of the last 50 years. Antioxidants are substances and/or built-in mechanisms the body uses to neutralize the harmful affects of free-radicals. Free radicals are highly reactive molecules that have the ability to do irreparable damage to cellular structures. Uncontrolled free radical aggression can disrupt normal metabolic functions of the cell.

How Free Radicals Are Formed

Free radicals are generated as by-products of normal metabolic cycles, as well as from cigarette smoke, environmental pollutants, exercise, poor dietary habits, and a host of other causes. Normally, the body can handle the amounts of free radicals it produces: however, when they begin to accumulate faster than they are neutralized, this can manifest itself in a number of different negative ways. Included among these are: lack of energy, fatigue, malaise, listlessness, colds, recurring yeast infections and a general decline in immune functions.

Antioxidants are now highly recommended as part of every nutritional program. In the following synopsis, we will take a look at a few of the more well-known supplements and their energy involvement as well as their antioxidant-producing capabilities.

Special Note: *Researchers have found what they believe to be a breakthrough to dwindling energy levels due to aging. Earlier, we learned that cells break down food molecules and that "ATP" is actually produced in the mitochondia of the cell. Scientists at John Hopkins University in Baltimore, MD have discovered that an enzyme called "ATP synthase," found in the mitochondria, spins around several times a second and helps recycle chemicals that help manufacture ATP.*

According to Dr. Peter Pedersen, Ph.D., if this enzyme didn't spin and recycle material, we would have to manufacture more than ½ of our body weight in ATP every day, to meet our energy needs.

These findings suggest that ATP synthase may be the actual site where free radical damage occurs, explaining why our energy levels begin to falter as we age, according to Dr. Pederson.

Bottom Line Here: Eat plenty of antioxidant-rich foods as well as use a high-quality antioxidant supplement.

Vitamins

Vitamin A — Is absolutely necessary for life. It builds immunity, protects the lungs against air pollution, and enhances visual purple, which is related to good eyesight. Recommended dose: 5000 IU (International Units). The popular vitamin Beta-Carotene is a pre-cursor to vitamin A. It is naturally converted by the body into vitamin A to meet dietary needs. Beta-carotene found abundantly in carrots is virtually non-toxic. Vitamin A from fish-liver oil has known toxicity levels at 50,000 I.U.'s (international units) and above when used long-term.

The Mighty B's

When you think of the B-vitamins, think of an orchestra. They work best when taken together. There are eleven members of the B-family. They help absorb and metabolize food to produce energy. They also help convert proteins, carbohydrates, and fats into fuel. In the brain, they help synthesize the mood-controlling chemicals.

Vitamin B1 — Thiamin. A deficiency can slow down the utilization of two brain chemicals: acetylcholine and serotonin (Neurology, 7; 81:691 Journal of Nut. Vol. 107. 10:77;1902.8). Without these brain chemicals, the transmission of nerve impulses is drastically hindered. Recommended dose: 1.5 mg.

B2 — Riboflavin. Also known as the 'youth vitamin'. Very beneficial in times of heightened stress. Recommended dose: 1.2-1.7 mg.

B3 — Niacin. Aids in promoting a healthy digestive and circulatory system. Increases energy by enhancing proper food utilization. Dose: 13-19 mg. daily.

B6 — Pyridoxine. Fats, carbohydrates, and all proteins metabolize more effectively in the presence of pyridoxine. It is also important to red blood cell formation. Suggested intake: 1.6-2 mg. daily.

B12 — Cobalamin.Commonly called the 'red vitamin' and one of the most well-known B vitamins, it is vital for its ability to form and regenerate red blood cells. Suggested dose: 2.2 mcg. (micrograms) daily.

Folic Acid — This vitamin has received much press recently due to its ability to prevent neural tube birth effects. More recent studies have cited it as a nutrient that can neutralize the artery-clogging effects of homocysteine. Homocysteine is a by-product created during the breakdown of certain amino acids. It is now known to be the major causative factor of heart disease. Folic acid also works with B12 in red blood cell formation. Recommended dosage: 18-21 mcg. (micrograms) Green leafy vegetables, carrots, liver, apricots and cantaloupe are excellent sources of folic acid.

Pantothenic Acid — This is Vitamin B-5. Called the anti-stress vitamin because it exerts a positive effect on the adrenal glands. As a coenzyme, it helps facilitate the release of energy from carbohydrates, fats, proteins and in the utilization of other vitamins.

Vitamin E — This vitamin is best known for its ability to insure heart health. Vitamin E helps promote circulation and has powerful antioxidant properties. Suggested dose, 30 IU daily.

Minerals: The Forgotten Heroes

Many of us fail to realize the full power and necessity of minerals. While vitamins are organic (living) substances, minerals are not. This implies that to some degree when conditions are right internally the body can make some vitamins. Humans are totally incapable of manufacturing any minerals.

Minerals, as stated, supply the electrical spark or energy that is necessary to keep the body's functions flowing. There is also one other important thing we tend to forget, and that is, without the presence of minerals as co-factors, vitamins are essentially worthless. In essence, without minerals, vitamins are incapable of doing their job.

Like vitamins, minerals function best when they are taken together rather than as separate supplements. The following summarizes the attributes of a few of them:

Chromium — One of the most important minerals, in terms of energy metabolism, because of its central role in potentiating insulin. Research has conclusively shown that all forms of chromium (chromium polynicotinate, chromium picolinate, chromium chloride, GTF chromium) can effectively balance insulin levels and normalize blood sugar levels. Suggested dose: 50mg daily.

Iron — One of the most well-known minerals. Builds blood, helps prevent anemia. Keeps cellular transport systems working well, and helps support the utilization of various enzymes within the krebs cycle. Dose range: 18 mg (women); 10 mg (men).

Special Note: *It is not advisable for men who consume meals balanced with 2000 calorie/day, to take additional iron supplements unless specified by a physician.*

Note: *If you are a male please do not overload your system with iron. Please stay within the recommended dose ranges. Additionally, I recommend* *taking iron in its citrate, gluconate, ferrous or fumarate form. These forms are less irritating on the stomach.*

Magnesium — This mineral is extremely important. It is necessary to the proper functioning of all energy dependent reactions. Magnesium is also necessary for ATP (our energy molecule) to be used for any of its energy transactions. Dose range: 400 mg. Best food sources of magnesium are figs, almonds, bananas, and dark green vegetables.

Phosphorus — Main mineral actively involved in ATP production, and also contributes to the metabolic energy potential. A deficiency will manifest itself in the form of low energy, vigor and stamina. Recommended dosage: 1.0 grams.

Potassium — Main mineral found in the cell. Helps maintain cell integrity and proper water balance. Vital to nerve function and the utilization of glucose and protein metabolism. Dose range: 1,600-2,000 mg.

Vanadium — An important mineral which supports the actions of chromium. Suggested dose: 10 to 15 mg daily.

Zinc — This mineral is known as the Master Mineral. It is involved with over 100 enzyme systems that are dependent on its presence. Zinc must also be present before glucose can be transported into the cells. Dose range: 15 mg.

Conclusion

With all the mounting evidence, many researchers, including myself, strongly advocate the addition of a vitamin and mineral supplement as part of your daily health regimen. As stated by J. Mark Davis of the Department of Exercise Science, at the University of South Carolina:

The often debilitating fatigue that accompanies viral or bacterial infections; recovery from injury or surgery, chronic fatigue syndrome, and depression almost certainly cannot be explained by a dysfunction with the muscle themselves.

I strongly recommend you consider the use of vitamins and minerals due to their overall metabolic as well as antioxidant capabilities.

Whole Food Factors

"Whole vegetables and fruits are composed of a considerable quantity of fibers. Within the interstices of these fibers are enclosed the atoms and molecules which are the essential nutritional elements we need. It is these atoms and molecules and their respective enzymes in the fresh-raw juices which aid the speedy nourishment of the cells and tissues, glands, organs, and every part of our body."

Dr. Norman W. Walker, D.S.C.
Health and Nutrition Advocate

The above statement by Dr. Walker may help to explain why the normal three meals a day may not be supplying you with all the energy you need. Also, for those of you who only eat one large meal and/or eat lots of fat-laden, processed foods, you can see why you feel drained.

Researchers now know that a whole line of supplements, as well as live fresh vegetable and fruit juices, contain that mighty green pigment, chlorophyll, responsible for converting the energy from the sun's rays to plants for our energy needs. The fantastic part in the use of these whole food factors is that, like everything else in nature, they are already packaged with an array of high-powered, energizing nutrients.

Since the rays of the sun send billions of atoms into plants activating enzymes that have the capability of converting inorganic (non-living) elements into organic (life-containing) elements, the use of these food factors (in supplements or liquid extracts, or as fresh fruit and vegetable juices) is highly recommended in today's environment. For the regeneration of all your cellular structures and body tissues, and ultimately your energy levels, the nourishment your cells receive must be in its live organic state.

While this book cannot cover the multitude of whole food factors and live juice therapy combinations available, we will take a look at a few of them.

Bee-pollen — Bee pollen is known as nature's miracle food. It is the male reproductive element of the flower. A bee brings a large amount of this pollen to the hive. It takes a bee around one hour to collect about 4,000,000 of these pollen grains. Locked up in these grains are powerful nutrients known to have the ability to regulate and stimulate metabolism by providing every nutrient known to man. Bee pollen works best on an empty stomach, 15-20 minutes before a meal.

Note: *Pollen is highly perishable and should be refrigerated or sealed in nitrogen. Fresh pollen is soft and has a sweet rather than a bitter after-taste.*

Kelp — Kelp is best known for its iodine content which supplies necessary nutrients for the proper working of the thyroid gland. The thyroid gland regulates your metabolic rate. When you consider that more than 59 elements are found in sea water solution, this magnifies the dynamic energy-producing capabilities of this whole food from the sea.

Liver — The liver is our detoxifying gland which protects us against toxins. When the liver isn't functioning properly, this affects our immunity, energy and general well-being. Desiccated (dried) liver extracts may help boost your energy levels as well as starve off anemia. Desiccated liver is not only a good source of food iron, it also contains large amounts of B-vitamins to help the body assimilate "heme", the organic form of iron.

Yeast — There are a number of yeast products available known as "nutritional yeast". Two popular ones are Brewer's Yeast and Torula Yeast. These yeasts naturally contain large amounts of B-vitamins (except B-12, which is usually added).Nutritional yeast also naturally contains as many as 16 of the amino acids, 17 or more vitamins and up to 14 minerals. When taken in conjunction with a B-complex nutritional supplement, this dynamic duo really packs a punch.

Blackstrap Molasses — Blackstrap molasses is a by-product of sugar refinement. Sugar cane naturally contains many vitamins and minerals. But in the process of making white sugar, these valuable nutrients are discarded. Gram for gram, blackstrap molasses contains more iron than any other food except pig liver and brewer's yeast. It contains about 5 times more calcium than milk, is loaded with B-vitamins and contains considerable amounts of minerals. As a pick-me-up or a good natural source of iron, blackstrap molasses will leave you feeling highly energized.

Green-Gold Food Factors

While there are literally hundreds of whole food combinations, supplements, extracts and powders, the following list represents some of the most popular products that are considered part of the "green gold" category, the superfoods of the next century. These supplements are rich in chlorophyll and will positively naturally revitalize, rejuvenate, and provide energy to the cells. I recommend you take some or all of these whole food extracts as a part of your daily supplement cycle, since they contain live organic substances which are vital to keep the human bioenergetic system functioning at its peak.

Old cells can be rejuvenated through this infusion of power from the sun, like getting a solar transfusion, on an ongoing basis. Daily usage may contribute to complete revitalization of your metabolic pathways.

Although not exhaustive, the following list represents many of these whole green foods:

- Alfalfa
- Celery juice
- Chlorella
- Chlorophyll
- Green Barley
- Fenugreek
- Green sprouts
- Kale
- Spirulina (Blue Green algae)
- Sorrel juice
- Watercress juice
- Wheat grass

Conclusion

Whole food extracts have an enormous potential to jump-start your energy levels as well as provide a flow of life-giving enzymes, vitamins, minerals and other food factors. They are "enzymatically alive", meaning that they are already energy-charged substances, and will provide the necessary components to energize existing out-of-balance metabolic pathways.

As stated by Dr. Norman Walker, except for accidents, all the repair and regeneration of our body must come from within. While losing a few pounds and exercising are steps in the right direction, incorporating whole food extracts (especially the green ones) into the diet will go a long way toward re-energizing a system depleted of its natural energy reserves.

Emerging Energizers

Exercise

Recent studies have shown that physical inactivity is a contributing factor to the onset of several chronic diseases. In fact, a sedentary life-style has been linked to 28% of all deaths from long-term chronic degenerative diseases. The American Heart Association has stated that physical inactivity is a major risk factor for contracting heart disease. Additionally, current research has revealed that there is increased endorphin activity from exercise. Endorphins are excitatory brain chemicals that energize the system. They play a major role in leaving you feeling refreshed and revitalized after a workout.

Based on the above and other related data, the Centers for Disease Control and Prevention suggest that every adult in the United States participate in thirty minutes or more of moderate intense physical activity of some sort every day of the week. These new guidelines have been mandated to complement, not replace, previous urging of at least twenty to thirty minutes of more vigorous, continuous aerobic exercise three to five times a week.

Regular moderate to vigorous exercise also has been shown to lower the risk of myocardial infarction (heart attack), stroke, hypertension (high blood pressure), type II diabetes and osteo-porosis. Recent surveys, however, indicate that adults in the US are active at the moderate level, and only 8% currently exercise at the more strenuous level, recommended for health benefits. Furthermore, nationwide surveys have revealed that 58% of Americans do not engage in any regular or leisure time physical activity.

If you are part of this last group, please consider the advise of Dr. Kenneth H. Cooper, known as the "fitness doctor". Dr. Cooper states:

Whatever the reason for exercising, if we want more energy we must give up more of the energy we already have. This assumption is rooted in the principles of aerobics, or requiring oxygen. Aerobic exercises force your heart to pump more blood and oxygen to the rest of your body. After a workout, even after your heart has returned to its pre-workout state, you feel more invigorated.

Detoxification

According to current thinking, constant bouts of fatigue for no apparent reasons could be due to what scientists call "xenobiotics". Xenobiotics is a term used to describe the alarming amount of pollutants, chemicals, and foreign toxins with which we are bombarded. In our era of high technology, we have had to contend with a number of chemicals that are foreign to living organisms. These by-products of the technologies used in our processed food chain have been linked to a variety of disorders. Alzheimer's, multiple sclerosis and chronic fatigue are examples. The problems associated with these maladies are metabolic in nature. It is clear that many of the foreign substances, such as heavy metals, including mercury from dental fillings; pesticides, artificial fertilizers, preservatives, flavoring agents, air and water born pollutants; all have the capability to interrupt normal metabolic cycles.

For this reason, it may be wise to consider some daily detoxification programs and/or specified cleansing regimes. By reducing the toxic elements in your system, you may be able to better control the quantity and duration of your short bouts with energy loss.

To get started, I would suggest you check with a health professional who specializes in natural detoxification programs. There are, however, a number of products (especially "detox" teas) which contain many herbs and other natural products known for their ability to cleanse vital organs such as the liver, colon, kidneys and the lymphatic system. You may want to consider the use of the following supplements:

- Astragalus — an immune booster
- Burdock Root — a natural liver/blood purifier
- Cranberry — cleans urinary tract
- Dandelion — a diuretic, flushes kidneys
- Echinacea — supports natural resistance
- Fiber — regulates digestive system
- Garlic — natural antibiotic
- Ginger — promotes good digestion
- Goldenseal — blood purifier
- Hawthorn — strengthens the heart
- Lactobacillus Acidophilus — supports intestinal health and cleanliness
- Lecithin — breaks down fat, cleanses liver
- Melatonin — a natural sleep aid
- Milk Thistle — liver cleanser
- Mullein — keeps lympathic system clean
- Red Clover — a strong blood cleanser
- Skullcap — helps promote sleep
- Yellow Dock — keeps bile active

Fasting

Fasting is one of the oldest methods used to cleanse internal organs and reduce toxic overload. While a short unsupervised fast can be beneficial, I do not recommend that they generally be done without the supervision of a qualified health professional.

In conclusion, the idea is to assist the body in its natural detoxification efforts. Keeping those eliminative organs working at their peak efficiency will go a long way toward boosting energy levels.

As stated by Lindsey Duncan, C.N., of the Home Nutrition Clinic of the Stars in Santa Monica, CA:

Similar to a septic system, the digestive and eliminative system needs to be cleaned in order to operate properly. Internal cleansing is one of the keys to a successful energy building program. When food is properly converted into nutrients, elevated levels of vitality are guaranteed.

Solving the Supplement Puzzle

In the world of supplements, the saying "One Size Fits All" does not apply. Like any well-planned diet and exercise program, you must also choose the right supplement to meet your changing needs. I would strongly suggest that you seek the services of a Certified Nutritionist (CN) or someone qualified to give you insight regarding the many products available. Additionally, once you have chosen a supplement to enhance your energy levels, keep the following factors in mind:

1. *Give yourself time.* These are food supplements and not drugs. In some cases it may take at least 30 days or so to get the nutrient properly circulating in the bloodstream. The point concerning consistency and timing was made by Dr. Barry Sears, in his book *"Enter The Zone"*. He states that every drug has a "therapeutic zone", and for it to be effective, you must maintain certain levels of it in the bloodstream. The same rule of thumb applies to food supplements.

2. *Take your supplements everyday.* In most cases, it will be preferably to take them with a meal.

Note: *Number 2 may not apply to herbs. Some herbs should be taken on cycles. For example, it is suggested that Echinacea be taken for not longer than 2 months, with a 2 month rest period thereafter before re-introducing the herb.*

3. As is the case with taking drugs, *follow the directions.* More is not always better. Stay within the established guidelines, as stipulated on your bottle.

4. *Liquids* — Do not take your supplements with coffee, tea or soda. Take with a full glass of water or fruit juice. Hot liquids (a misconception) do not activate the actions of the ingredients.

5. *Dependency* — These are natural food supplements and you don't have to worry about becoming addicted to these natural dietary supplements. However, you also shouldn't depend on these substances to cover poorly planned diet and exercise regimens. They are designed to augment your efforts, not replace them.

6. *Selection* — Supplements are not created equal. Some are stronger than others, and have full label disclosure of its ingredients. Look for expiration dates. If the company doesn't list one on its label, find one that does. Also check to see if the product is loaded with inert binders and fillers. These substances have no medicinal value, neither do preservatives, or sugars.

7. *Experimentation* — As stated in the opening caption, in the world of supplements, one size doesn't fit all. The great thing about natural supplementation is that it gives you the ability to experiment within limits. It may take you a while to find and even determine which combination or group of products are just right for you. I suggest that people use their intelligence in finding the right combination. Also be patient — it may take natural supplements a little longer to work. In the long run, however, they assist in modulating (balancing) metabolic function — this is what you want!

Your health and sense of well-being should be your final test in determining how well a product is working for you.

There are literally thousands of substances being researched as possible adjuncts to resolving the current human energy crisis. The list of new substances is extensive, as cited below, with reports coming in everyday citing the benefits of many other new compounds:

Mustard seeds	Red wine	Omega 3 fish oils
Chinese gooseberry	Medium chain tri-glycerides (MCT)	Dahlulin
Kola nuts	Cijwi	Glutathione
Guarana	Evening Primrose	Water (H2O)
DHEA	Inosine	Licorice Root
Green Kamut	Chromium	Peppermint
Wild Yams	Black Cohosh	Ribose

Recommendations

It is imperative that careful consideration be made in relationship to individual needs, lifestyles and age before incorporating an herb, vitamin or accessory supplement into your dietary regimen. Due to the massive conglomeration of natural energizers and supplements, this author suggest building a supplement program which focuses on:

- Daily Needs (long term usage)
- Digestive Needs (long term usage)
- Metabolic Needs (intermittent)
- Energy Needs (intermittent)
- Short Term Needs (minimal usage)
- Experimental (toward the short term)

In the next chapter, "Energy, Aging and Immunity", we will take a look at how aging affects your energy levels and how you can prepare for this stage of life to insure that your full energy potential does not diminish or falter. The overall goal of this chapter is to take a much more extensive look at "antioxidants" and their role in neutralizing the harmful effects of ravenous molecules called free radicals.

Chapter Six

ENERGY, AGING AND IMMUNITY

"Over time, various age changes, as gerontologists call them, exert massive influence. But at any given moment, aging accounts for only 1 percent per year of the total change taking place inside your body. In other words, 99 percent of the energy and intelligence that you are composed of is untouched by the aging process."

Dr. Deepak Chopra, M.D.
Ageless Body-Timeless Mind

It is a misconception that aging is a disease and that it inevitably causes deterioration of our immune system and energy levels. As expressed by Dr Deepak Chopra, 99 percent of the energy and intelligence that we are composed of is untouched by the aging process. If this is true,

- Why do energy levels seem to diminish as we get older?
- Why does immunity seem to decline with the aging process?
- What causes the body to age?
- Can I slow this process down?
- What changes are occurring as I age?
- Do these changes occur gradually or do they start spontaneously later in life?

- If aging accounts for only 1 percent annual decrease in my potential energy and intelligence, does my internal system remain youthful?

Aging, according to the late Dr. Carlton Fredericks, Ph.D., a pioneer in the application of nutritional supplements, although linked to a number of degenerative conditions, doesn't necessarily imply causation of these conditions. In other words, loss of energy and decreased immunity may not be a direct result of aging.

This is the focus of chapter six. We also will take a look at Dr. Chopra's contention that aging has little to do with the destruction of your energy potential. Additionally, in this chapter, we will take a look at the real cause of this degenerative process.

The Invisible Hand of Nature

As stated earlier, just as people are born with the potential to grow to a particular height, they're also born with a genetically-determined energy potential. Furthermore, humans have an inborn cycle of events that continually assists the body's internal mechanisms that produce energy. Dr. William Lee reminds us, however, that although nature has provided much, in some ways, nature can be cruel. According to Dr. Lee, some scientists believe that, because survival of the species is the dominant force in all organisms, including humans, they function at their best while young. Once they have passed on their genes to the next generation, nature hasn't much use for them any more and hasn't bothered to provide for long term optimum maintenance of the system.

Dr. Lee also maintains that after age twenty-six or so, the production of hormones, enzymes, and other protective substances our bodies need to insure survival, vigor, fun, and good health is gradually reduced. Dr. Stuart Berger, M.D., author of *Forever Young*, assesses nature's control of this decline with the following statement:

> *Perhaps the most profound changes happen where you can't see or hear them, deep within your cellular and organ systems. In virtually every niche and cranny of your body, aging means the power and strength of your organs and cells are gradually waning.*

The Great Metabolism Shift

Dr. Berger claims that somewhere around the beginning of your fourth decade, your energy furnaces start to burn differently. During this time, nature begins to leave you with an extra layer of fat. As fat increases, you also lose lean muscle mass. Muscle is a highly metabolic tissue; pound for pound, it burns five times as many calories as most other body tissues. The addition of ten pounds of muscle in the body can burn 600 calories per day. People would have to run six miles per day seven days per week to burn the same number of calories. In fact, ten extra pounds of muscle can burn a pound of fat in one week, which is 52 pounds of fat per year.

What this translates into is the accumulation of extra unwanted pounds which can have a dramatic impact on existing energy levels as well as an overall decline in health. The rate at which and how efficiently the body burns calories is known as the basal metabolic rate. The rate at which the body utilizes these calories for energy is of vital importance to maintaining your energy potential on a daily basis. Dr. Berger also maintains that to stay young and vital for as long as possible, you need some idea of what really happens as a body grows older. Some of the changes you can expect as nature throttles down your internal engine are:

- A drop of almost three percent, every decade, of your basal metabolic rate;
- A reduction in the amount of oxygen that is transported into the cells;
- A change in the body's ability to absorb nutrients;
- A gradual decline in the body's immune response;
- A rise in the blood level of abnormal proteins. One of these proteins, rheumatoid factors, is implicated in arthritic inflammation of the joints;
- A drop from six to three quarts of air in your lung capacity with each breath;
- A drop in the pumping of the heart from a high of almost four quarts of blood a minute at age 25 to only two and a half quarts at age 65.

Keeping Your Foot On The Pedal

As you can see, nature has not given you a reserve battery for long-term peak operation of many internal mechanisms. However, you have the ability to recharge and clean your current battery to help offset this invisible hand of nature.

New reports show that the air we breathe, the food we eat, the water we drink, everyday stress, and even our own body's normal use of oxygen create toxic molecules called free radicals that can wreak havoc on our immune systems and our cells. In turn, we age faster, our energy levels decline, and we may develop many chronic health problems. To help offset this invisible or "silent" decline by nature, many health and medical professionals are recommending that you pay careful attention to your daily intake of antioxidants via food consumption and vitamin supplementation.

It is important to note here that consumption of organic foods doesn't totally shield one from free radical production. Free radicals are formed during normal metabolic processes. The goal, however, is to minimize their formation, assisted by the consumption of fresh organic foods.

Antioxidants: The Youth Nutrients

Wilfred Trotler (1877 – 1939), the consulting surgeon to the University College Hospital in London and Honorary Surgeon to the King (1928 – 32) stated that, "the most powerful antigen known to man is a new idea." That idea or scientific fact has arrived with the discovery of the neutralizing effects antioxidants have on free radicals and their ability to enhance the immune response.

The most compelling new studies come from such prestigious research centers as the National Cancer Institute (NCI), the National Institute on Aging, Johns Hopkins University, Harvard University and the American Heart Association. With each new study, we find exciting new breakthroughs on antioxidants isolated from fruits and vegetables and how they function within our bodies' cellular and tissue systems.

Antioxidants and the Immune System

There has been much debate concerning the supplementation of one's diet as a preventive measure against disease. The late Dr. Richard H. Follis of the Nutritional Control Laboratory for Anatomical Pathology and Research has noted that the most important point to realize in consideration of the naturally occurring deficiency diseases in man, is that these diseases result from a lack of multiple nutrients rather than the deficiency of a single essential nutrient.

We know that specific fruits, vegetables and other plant foods carry hundreds of protective compounds called phytonutrients that protect us against the devastating effects of free radicals. As study after study emerges, we see how antioxidant — rich phytonutrients help to enhance natural immunity, slow down and even reverse some of the damage aging can cause. In practical terms, the powerful attributes of these substances (antioxidants) can have a significant impact in helping you to maintain and manage your full energy potential and immunity, as well as slowing down the negative internal aspects of aging.

Dr. Robert Willix, M.D., states that antioxidants are the most important medical discovery in the last fifty years. Dr. Willix insists that this assumption is based on the fact that many viruses and bacteria that cause diseases like colds, smallpox, typhoid, tuberculosis and so forth have been eradicated and/or are treatable. Most of the great successes of modern medicine can be traced back to Louis Pasteur's germ theory of disease. However, according to Dr. Willix, germs are no longer the big killers of our time. The big killers are cancer, stroke, and heart disease. Our bodies are weakened by allergies, arthritis, headaches and chronic fatigue which are not caused by germs but by free radical damage. Dr. Willix gives an overview of the importance of antioxidants and their overall capabilities in the following synopsis:

*There are two aspects of the so-called "aging process." It's very important for you to understand the difference, **because one of them can be controlled or reversed.** The part of the aging* *process that can't be controlled involves the "biological clocks" that are built into our genes. Changes like puberty, menopause and male pattern baldness are genetically programmed. In general they can't be controlled yet. But most people don't die of these genetically programmed changes. They die of cancer, stroke and heart disease largely caused by free-radical damage. This is the part of the aging process that you can control or reverse.*

Dr. Betty Kamen, Ph.D., an award winning journalist, maintains that perhaps the most important role of antioxidant nutrients is to help prevent proteins in cell membranes from being damaged. Proteins are the large, complex and specialized molecules that actually control the functioning of important cell membranes. The membranes let nutrients in, send waste products out, and block entry of toxins or viral invaders.

Know Your Antioxidants

In recent years, scientific evidence has been pouring in on the benefits of antioxidants. Dr. David Perlmutter, a well-known health professional, believes that we are experiencing a carotene revolution. Think of this revolution as a color war. The antioxidant army consists of a host of brilliant green, yellow, orange, blue, red, purple and violet vegetables and fruits, while the cancer army consists of a ragtag collection of brown and gray cells. Dr. Kamen, whom I spoke of earlier, contends that the best natural sources of antioxidants tend to be the greenest and fastest growing plants because sunlight, which is high-energy solar radiation, is being used to drive the photosynthesis reaction. The U.S. Department of Agriculture and the U.S. Department of Health and Human Services recommend that we get three to five servings from these food groups, meaning the bright colored fruits and vegetables, everyday.

To get a clear picture of which groups of food have a positive or negative effect on the immune response, please see appendix D located in the rear of this book. To cultivate, manage, and maintain your full energy potential, it is critical that you become a "food detective", and continuously investigate how foods and their antioxidant capabilities affect your ability to mount and maintain a strong immune response.

Dr. Earl Mindell, Ph.D., R.P.H., states that his top four antioxidants are what he calls the "ACES". Vitamin A (Beta Carotene), Vitamin C, Vitamin E and Selenium. The best food sources of Vitamin A and Beta Carotene, sometimes called provitamin A, are such colored vegetables as carrots, beets, yams and squash. The best food sources of Vitamin C are fruits and vegetables such as greens and sprouts. Some excellent food sources of Vitamin E are whole grains, nuts and seeds. Selenium, a trace mineral which is often lacking in modern diets as a result of its deficiency in soils, is found in the bran germ of grains and also in vegetables such as broccoli, onions and tomatoes.

Antioxidants and Vitamin Co-Factors

The antioxidant researchers Kronhausen, Kronhausen and Demopoulous state that "if you observe three basic rules, you will "unleash" the "power" and "force" of several micronutrients (nutrients needed in small amounts), magnified by the dominant power of antioxidants and vitamin co-factors". Those three rules are:

1. Take only pure pharmaceutical (USP) grade antioxidants and vitamin co-factors with no contaminants or additives. (Author's Note: Food-based supplements are also viable sources.)
2. Take micronutrients in recommended doses only — high enough to prevent free-radical damage, but not so high as to cause toxicities.
3. Take them only in a broad combination or spectrum, so that they can work together and recycle each other for maximum effectiveness.

Technically, number three above is referred to as synergism. Synergism takes into account the interaction of various nutrients and their combined effect versus a single nutrient alone. The right way to take antioxidants and their co-factors is as a part of a spectrum of mutually complementary micronutrients. Even the late Nobel Prize-winning chemist Linus Pauling, a longtime advocate of high doses of Vitamin C, recommended that Vitamin C be taken along with other vitamins for best results.

Kronhausen, Kronhausen and Demopoulous have also formulated a fundamental rule for anyone wishing to supplement their diet with antioxidants, vitamins and their co-factors. Their rule states that:

If you take Vitamin C, you must also take Vitamin E. If you take Vitamin E, it's best to also take Beta Carotene and glutathione. And if you take any of these antioxidants, you must take high doses of the B vitamins to provide a steady stream of electrons and hydrogen to reconstitute the antioxidants that would otherwise be sacrificed as they do their job of quenching free radicals.

The Study of Free Radical Damage

Free radical reactions have been investigated as possible factors in the aging process since the late 1950's, when Dr. Denham Harman first formulated the free radical theory of aging. Dr. Stuart M. Berger, M.D., states "that researchers are quite unequivocal concerning free radicals, maintaining that 99 percent of the free radicals are the basis for aging." Kronhausen, Kronhausen and Demopoulous also agree that the study of free radicals and the damage that their uncontrolled activity can do to all the organs in the body has led for the first time in medical history to a unified theory of disease and aging. According to the above health professionals, free radical pathology (the study of disease processes associated with free radical activity) has given us a better understanding, not only of such degenerative diseases as atherosclerosis and cancer, but also of the aging process, the shrinking of the internal organs, and the mental deterioration that often accompanies it. Furthermore, free radical pathology plays a part in immune system suppression and the body's resulting susceptibility to infectious diseases and depressed energy levels.

The Composition of Free Radicals

A free radical is not a living thing like a virus or a bacteria. Viruses, bacteria and the cells in your body are made up of molecules. A free radical is much smaller than that. It is a single reactive molecule. These predators are like ravenous molecular sharks, and last only a millionth of a second. The problem with a free radical is that it contains an oxygen atom with a missing electron. A free radical can't rest until it replaces that missing electron and, generally, the only way it can get an electron is by taking a bite out of another molecule, thus causing a chain of reactions that can:

- Damage cellular structures
- Depress natural metabolics (energy producing cycles)
- Inactivate enzyme systems
- Cause hardening of the arteries
- Damage blood vessels
- Accelerate the aging process
- Contribute toward cancer growth
- Depress the immune system

Understanding Free Radical Aggression

Dr. Earl Mindell states that antioxidants are substances that help neutralize the damage of oxidation in the body. We can think of oxidation as similar to what happens to metal when it rusts, or to an apple when it turns brown. Unstable oxygen molecules go to war in the body grabbing on to other cells in their attempt to become stable.

The bio-chemists Pearson and Shaw also argue that the tiniest killers today aren't viruses, but a type of indiscriminate reactive molecule or molecule fragment called a free radical. The above researchers contend that since our life depends on very careful control of the chemical reactions within us, free radicals can be deadly. Studies have shown that free radicals attack and alter cellular enzymes, the protein-derived catalysts that speed all metabolic processes. The damaged enzyme is inactivated, which slows or halts all processes dependent on the enzyme (the liberation of energy). Additionally, free radicals activate dormant (inactive) enzymes that in turn cause tissue damage and disease, such as emphysema, or can release neurotoxins that affect nerve and brain functions.

Pearson and Shaw, however, remind us that some of these free radicals are necessary participants in certain normal metabolic reactions. Accordingly, the body supplies enzymes which control free radicals so that they don't escape to do damage. The enzymes, superoxide dismutase (SOD) and glutathione peroxidase are two of these free radical control substances made in your body. Without these enzymes, you would quickly die. In fact, all air-breathing life on our planet must have such enzymes to survive.

What's Wrong With Oxidation?

Oxygen is a toxin as well as a necessity for most animals and plants. Even in the course of normal metabolism involving ordinary amounts of oxygen, harmful free radicals are created. According to Dr. Betty Kaman, Ph.D., despite the fact that oxidation is one of the most fundamental and necessary biochemical reactions, not all oxidation is desirable. In fact Dr. Kaman claims that oxidation of the wrong substances at the wrong time can have a devastating effect on health. Dr. Kaman cites the following reasons why excessive oxidation wreaks havoc on the immune system:

- Oxidation can render basic cellular level immune responses inoperable;
- Oxidation can also damage fatty acids by filling in the "unsaturated" locations in the chain of atoms. In other words, a polyunsaturated fat may become partially saturated through the oxidation process;
- Oxidation may cause cross-linking. Here long-protein molecules that make up skin, tendons, and arteries sometimes bond to each other in undesirable ways after oxidation damage. The immediate result is usually a significant

loss of flexibility and elasticity. The long term result is wrinkled skin, stiff joints and inelastic arteries.

Energy and Immunity

If you want to insure that you live a long, healthy and vibrant life, nothing is more crucial than the proper functioning of your immune system. Dr. Stuart Berger describes the overall importance of a strong immune response in the following statement:

This network of blood, cells, antibodies and chemicals is your body's protection against the diseases that age us all. It fights germs, from common bacteria to exotic parasites to the deadliest viruses. It is also your sole guardian against the malignant, often deadly, growth of cancer. Your immune system is all that stands between you and diseases that can sap your energy, threaten your life, and make your body weak and infirm (not stable) many years too soon.

What's The Right Dose

Currently, governmental agencies have not established RDAs for these powerful neutralizing substances, (antioxidants). The Alliance for Aging Research, a non-profit organization funded by philanthropic organizations, pharmaceutical companies and other contributors has urged the Food and Drug Administration to recommend how much Beta Carotene, Vitamin C, Vitamin E and other antioxidants we should take. A panel of experts from the Alliance has recommended these dosages:

1. 250 to 1,000 mg/day of Vitamin C. Current RDA (Recommended Daily Allowance) is 100 mg/day for smokers and 60 mg/day for others.
2. 100 to 400 iu/day of Vitamin E. Current RDA is 30 iu.
3. 17,000 to 50,000 iu/day of Beta Carotene. No RDA has been established for this nutrient.

The panel cited a number of studies which supported their recommendations on antioxidants. One of these, published in the *Journal of the National Cancer Institute*, found that almost 30,000 adults in Linxian, China, who received Beta Carotene and Vitamin E had reduced risks of cancer.

The Harvard School of Public Health studies, published in the New England Journal of Medicine in June 1993, showed a reduced risk of heart disease in both men and women who took Beta Carotene and Vitamin E. (1993)

As the evidence continues to mount, researchers are conducting investigations of global proportions to assess the long term benefits of these dynamic, and "youth" oriented nutrients. Many other nutrients such as zinc, copper, amino acids, coenzyme Q10, grape-seed extract, garlic, superoxide dismutase (SOD), B-complex vitamins, quercetin and a host of herbal and medicinal plant preparations or extracts, are also being touted as having possible antioxidant properties.

Negating The Invisible Hand of Nature

As discussed earlier, we now know that nature begins to throttle down our internal engine around the age of 26. Chronological age, which represents your age since birth, may not be entirely representative of your current biological age. Many health experts today believe that every individual has the power, not only to increase their energy levels, but also to control how their internal systems age. Current data has substantiated earlier claims by researchers that antioxidants have a profound affect on minimizing, as well as slowing down, the negative aspects of aging.

Your Antioxidant Profile

To get an accurate gauge on your current need to incorporate antioxidants into your daily food or supplement regimen please take the quiz found in appendix C at the end of this book. After taking this "antioxidant profile" quiz, you'll be able to make a subjective (non-conclusive) decision concerning your real biological age, and what adjustments you may need to make.

Conclusions

As stated by the late Dr. Carlton Fredericks, Ph.D., "the concept of aging should not be used as an excuse for a degenerative disease based on correlation." Correlation implies that a particular degenerative disease may go hand in hand with aging, but according to Dr. Fredericks, it does not prove causation. In this case, the depressed immunity, and loss of energy do not occur as a direct result of aging.

Current research has established a clear link to diminished energy levels and decreased immunity as a direct result of long-term chemical reactions that have gone astray. However, scientists have also confirmed that these imperfect reactions can be controlled and/or neutralized to some degree by individual intervention. In essence, chronological aging is immaterial if you maintain a healthy lifestyle. In fact, according to Dr. Lawrence B. Slobody, M.D., author of *The Golden Years: A 12 Step Anti-Aging Plan for a Longer, Healthier and Happier Life*, antioxidants help keep us vibrant and in good health by protecting as well as detoxifying our bodies.

Dr. Slobody goes on to say that recent research has confirmed that the application of antioxidants via nutritional and supplemental sources are key ways to get these anti-free radical substances.

As stated earlier by Dr. Robert Willix, antioxidants are the most important medical discovery in the last 50 years. It would be wise to learn as much as you can about these dynamic substances. More importantly, incorporating them into your daily nutritional and supplemental regimen may be the most important thing you can do in reaching and maintaining your full energy potential.

In the next chapter we will take a closer look at you and your individual lifestyle. From that lifestyle we will be able to determine which areas in your life could be contributing to your inability to realize your full energy potential. In essence we will be looking at, **"Your Individual Energy-Fatigue Profile"**

Health and Energy Ought to Flow From the Way We Live.

Paraphrase from Dr. Andrew Weil, M.D.
American Health, May, 1998

Chapter Seven

YOUR INDIVIDUAL FATIGUE PROFILE

"How we respond to the common and uncommon events and circumstances of our lives largely determines how healthful or destructive these situations will be. As the Roman Emperor Marcus Aurelius pointed out nearly 2,000 years ago, if you are distressed by anything external, the pain is not due to the thing itself but your estimate of it. This you have the power to revoke at any time."

Paul M. Insel and Walton T. Roth
Core Concepts In Health

Until recently, modern western medical science treated the body and the mind as two separate and independent entities. It looked at physical health as unrelated to psychological well-being. New medical research, however, has revealed that "psychological" factors can cause disease and influence energy levels. In fact, scientists now know that as certain perceived or real psychological factors mount, disease states (both physical and mental) as well as potential energy stores or levels become problematic.

One of these key factors that has gotten a lot of attention over the last decade is stress. The first wave of systematic stress research, dominating the field in the 30's, 40's, and early 50's, was the "psychosomatic movement". This branch labored to define those personality types most likely to contract ulcers, heart trouble,

143

migraines, arthritis and other specific ills. One of the best known investigations of the relationship between disease and susceptibility to disease was the research conducted by Meyer Friedman and Ray Rosenman in the 1950's. From their research emerged the type "X' personality (aggressive and fiercely competitive) which showed a high correlation to stress and the onset of various disease states.

Subsequent research conducted at the Harvard Medical School, Tufts University of Medicine, the Linus Pauling Institute, Carleton University (in Ottawa Canada) and at the University of Toronto have confirmed a direct link to stress as a major contributing factor to decreased immune function and the onset of chronic fatigue. In fact, medical experts today claim that the deciding factor in precipitating the extreme unrelenting form of fatigue known as the chronic fatigue syndrome" is stress.

Because of the concern of an increasing number of individuals afflicted with the above syndrome, emphasis today is focused on the physical and chemical pathways in which stress manifests itself within the body. Much of how and what health professionals know about the body's adaptive responses to stress is credited to an eminent endocrinologist and biochemist named Hans Hugo Selye.

Selye and Stress

Hans Selye is known as the father of stress research. This Austrian born scientist is credited with establishing a clear link between stress and the onset of chronic degenerative diseases. Based on his research findings, Selye made the following remarks:

We have learned that the body possesses a complex machinery of self-regulating checks and balances. These are remarkably effective in adjusting ourselves to virtually anything that can happen to us in life. But often this machinery does not work perfectly. Sometimes our responses are too weak, and they do not offer adequate protection. At other times they are too strong, and we actually hurt ourselves by our own excessive reactions to stress.

When and how the body interprets various stress responses and the overall adjustments it makes to constant internal and external changes is what Selye called the "GAS" (General Adaptation System) or "Stress Syndrome". In general, Selye defined stress as the common denominator of all the body's adaptive reactions (the non-specific response of the body to any demand). Demands could be pleasant and curative (eu stress) or unpleasant and disease producing (distress).

The key question however concerning this general adaptive system is:

Can this defense mechanism be hindered or impaired in its operation, and what effect does this have on our inborn energy potential?

The general adaptation syndrome (GAS) according to Selye develops in three stages. They are:
- The alarm reaction
- Resistance (or adaptive) stage, and
- Exhaustion

Alarm

This is the fight or flight response triggered by a perceived threat to the organism. During the course of this initial phase of arousal, your body perceives a stressor, something new or unusual that seems to present danger.

Norman Shealy, M.D., director of the Shealy Institute for Comprehensive Health Care in Springfield, Missouri, and a pioneer in the concept of "Transcutaneous Electrical Nerve Stimulation" (Tens), maintains that one of the least understood and recognized aspects of stress is that stress includes physical, chemical, emotional and electromagnetic factors. According to Dr. Shealy, the major stressors can be categorized as follows:

PHYSICAL
- Inactivity
- Toxins
- Inadequate light
- Allergens
- Temperature extremes
- Trauma

CHEMICAL
- Sugar
- Infection
- Nutrition imbalance
- Nicotine
- Caffeine
- Alcohol

EMOTIONAL	ELECTROMAGNETIC

EMOTIONAL
- Fear
- Anger
- Guilt
- Anxiety
- Depression
- Pain
- Inadequate sleep

ELECTROMAGNETIC
- Automobiles
- Refrigerators
- Television
- Computers
- Computer printers
- Airplanes
- Fluorescent lights

As mentioned by Dr. Shealy, the effects of the above stressors are ordinarily handled in the body by a balancing mechanism called "homeostasis". However, as reported by Dr's. Earle Richard and David Imrie of the Canadian Institute of Stress, regardless of the kind of stressor, your stress reaction is the same, as shown in figure 7.1. This illustration describes the varied physiological changes that occur during this alarm stage. The more this alarm goes off, the greater the negative impact will be to your existing energy potential or reserves.

Figure 7.1: The Body's Response To Stress

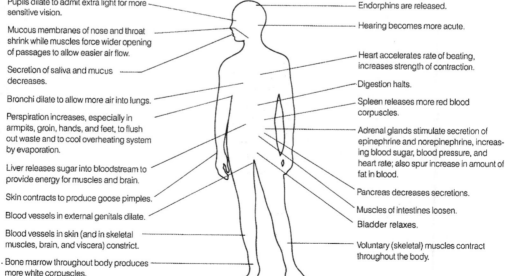

Figure 7.1 Source: Paul M. Insel and Walton T. Roth, *Core Concepts In Health*, Mayfield Publishing, Mountain View, CA, 1988, p. 27.

These chemical and electrical changes in your body are controlled by your hypothalamus. The hypothalamus is located at the base of the brain, and regulates the majority of the body's unconscious processes, such as temperature, heart rate, water balance, breathing, and blood pressure. It's job is to maintain homeostasis, the body's internal balance.

It is during this alarm state that the body shifts gears and enters phase two in an attempt to regain control, "the resistance stage".

Resistance

This is the stage in which the body attempts to adapt to (and compensate for) the physiological changes occurring from the alarm stage. It is an attempt to regain homeostasis.

Special Note: *The 19th century French Physiologist Claude Bernard, of the College de France in Paris, taught that one of the most characteristic features of all living beings is their ability to maintain the constancy of their internal milieu (internal environment of the body) despite changes in their surroundings. Walter B. Cannon, the famous Harvard physiologist, subsequently called this innate power "homeostasis".*

Balance is the Key

Dr. Phil Nuernberger (*Freedom From Stress*) contends that healthy nonstress functioning is represented by a balance between the alarm and resistance stage. This can take the form of a dynamic balance, constantly adjusting back and forth in a seesaw fashion, as represented by the dotted lines in figure 7.2.

Balance and the Autonomic Nervous System

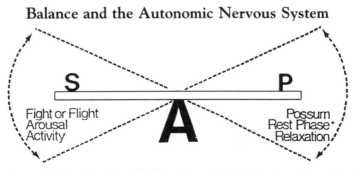

Figure 7.2 Source: *Freedom From Stress*, Phil Nuernberger, PH.D., Himalayan International Institute of Yoga Science and Philosophy, Honesdale, PA, 1981, p. 72.

Special Note: *Although the body seeks to maintain balance here, complete balance or a state of constancy of the internal milieu is not fully realized during this stage.*

Dr. Nuernberger goes on to say that "as long as the pattern of activity remains balanced (shifting back and forth in a fluid or dynamic pattern) there is no stress." Consequently periods of arousal (or activity) are healthy and nonstressful as long as they are balanced by periods of "inhibition" (relaxation and rest). However, if a state of inhibition is not balanced by activity, this can also become dysfunctional, resulting in energy loss causing lethargy and depression.

Balance and Homeostasis

Researchers now know that stable homeostasis does not totally occur between the two divisions (alarm and resistance) as represented by the "solid" line in figure 7.2. At this point the body is relaxed, but there is always the threat of a new stressor emerging. How well you are able to adapt to a new stressor will determine how long and how well you will maintain homeostasis. In this state, however, the mind is alert. This is an extremely healthy state in which there is no stress, although a great deal of physical and mental activity can be accomplished during it.

Note: It is this internal balance and the diminishing effects of prolonged stressors that constantly reduce our threshold for a new stressor, as cited by Selye. The significance of this statement lies in the fact that by the time you have adapted to three or four stressors, or even hundreds, it may take less than half as much of a new stressor to cause an alarm reaction.

In the state of alarm reaction, if the body doesn't regain homeostasis and is constantly adjusting to unresolved stress reactions, exhaustion sets in.

Exhaustion and Stress Energy

This stage occurs when the threat or stressor has gone away or subsided. This state also occurs when you run out of available "stress energy". Your body's energy comes from the food you eat but the way you experience this energy, for instance, or how available it is when you need it is primarily due to a bodily process called the "stress reaction". The stress reaction mobilizes and channels your available energy to meet any challenge you face.

Whatever the stressful situation, real or imagined, your body initially reacts and interprets it as an emergency. In essence, your energy levels and how you maintain them is largely a result of "adaptation".

The Key Question and Adaptive Energy

Earlier, a key question was asked concerning the general adaptive system and its various stages, which was:

Does this defensive mechanism ever stop working and what effect would this have on our inborn energy potential?

Well, during the exhaustion phase, if the arousal continues without effective adaptation, the body's attempt to create balance, as well as the effects of the arousal itself, lead to a depletion of reserve fuel (your energy potential), and you begin to suffer with bouts of exhaustion or chronic fatigue. In this state, physiological systems begin to break down and energy levels are constantly depleted. As expressed by Dr. Bernard Jensen, Ph.D., a Holistic Health Healer and Educator:

"The first day of your life that you experience less energy, less vitality and less mental power, is the first day of your impending illness."

Hans Selye compared each person's supply of adaptive energy to a nation's deposits of oil. Once you have summoned it up and burned it, it is gone. Han's Selye's "General Adaptation Syndrome", which depicts the time level the body stays in and responds to an acute (short-term stressor) or the response time to a prolonged stress reaction has been used to evaluate how well the body adapts to stressful situations.

Note: The Key Question Answered

If there is no relief from the exhaustion stage, the resultant stress on the physiological systems will lead to the "death" of the organism. In other words, in a state of constant arousal (or what is referred to as stress), the organism literally wears itself out!

Building A Model Of Fatigue

William Ascher, author of *Forecasting: An Appraisal For Policy-Makers and Planners* (1985) stated "because of past failures to foresee or acknowledge trends, that many problems we face today seem worse than they might otherwise have been". Conversely, Harold D. Lasswell (Ford Foundation, Professor Emeritus of Law and Social Science) formulated an important theory called "assumption drug". The significance of this theory and its application here, is that it proposes identifying a series of each problems that can be overcome by creating organized scenarios of each situation while looking for solutions to improve it.

To assess the likelihood of producing more power from your own inborn energy potential, you need to look at your current lifestyle. There may be certain stressors that have become part of your daily existence, that could be contributing to your current fatigue. According to Dr. Dharma Singh Khalsa, M.D., author of *Brain Longevity*, many of us do not understand the importance of stress management. Dr. Khalsa states that patients think the word stress refers to an outside force that causes them to feel tension." According to Dr. Khalsa, that's not stress, though—that's a 'stressor'.

Stress itself can be defined as the feeling that can result from a stressor. This distinction as cited by Dr. Khalsa may seem insignificant, but is important. Important because it means that if you don't perceive a stressor as stressful, then it's not one, as stated in the opening remarks of this chapter by the researchers, Insel and Roth.

To determine the current impact certain stressors and your response to them may have on your health and energy levels, please refer to Appendix D, Your Individual Fatigue Profile, located in the rear of this book. This exercise, known as *The Brain Longevity Stress Impact Index,* was formulated by Dr. Khalsa, whose specialty is in research concerning the causes of cognitive (something known or perceived) decline and brain longevity.

Although there have been many stress indexes developed by scientists over the years, such as the Holmes-Rahe Index, which ranks stressors on a scale of one to 100, many of them do not take into account the concept of 'perception'. This is important, since no two persons react the same to any given stressor. *The Brain Longevity Stress Impact Index* has been designed to account for a individual's probable perception of a given stressor and its impact on long-term health and "dynamia". As a point of reference here, dynamia is defined as having vital energy or the ability to combat disease.

Once you have finished, you should review your answers and analyze your score. This exercise can help you pinpoint crucial areas in your life that need attention to move you toward a more energized stated of existence.

This exercise can also be repeated over time (as necessary) to assess the direction in which you are headed, as you take steps to address your problem areas. Remember, identifying the causes of your fatigue is the first step toward eliminating them.

"Stress is a term used mostly in physics to mean strain, pressure or force on a system. When used in relation to the body cells, it describes the effects of the body reaction to a stressor, meaning a fairly predictable arousal of psychophysiological (mind-body) systems that, if prolonged, can fatigue or damage the system to the point of malfunction and disease."

Dr. Daniel A. Girdano, Ph.D.
Dr. George S. Everely, Jr., Ph.D.
Dr. Dorothy E. Dusek, Ph.D.
Controlling Stress and Tension
A Holistic Approach

Conclusions

Based on current data, there seems to be a strong correlation between one's ability to handle stress and diminished energy levels. Identifying just what those stressors are can have an immediate (positive) impact on energy maintenance and the preservation of health. Additionally, becoming aware of your individual personality type and its susceptibility toward perpetuating disease states is crucial to sustaining long-term health and energy levels.

Furthermore, your perception of stress and/or the significance of an individual stressor, plays a major role in conserving "stress energy". In other words, your ability to adapt to any given situation will largely determine how much energy you have or don't have. Take your time to analyze your score and results. Do not badger yourself if you feel the results are poor or need immediate attention. This moment should be viewed as an opportunity and a look toward the future. Look beyond your fatigue and envision how you can start making the necessary changes that will get you back on the right track.

Start slow and do not try and make across-the-board adjustments. Give yourself some time, and begin to make gradual changes. This process should be an evolution, not an all-out revolution.

Think big, but most of all, take the full responsibility for making and following thru on the changes needed. In the end, a new, more energetic, and healthier you will emerge!

Chapter Eight

MANAGING YOUR ENERGY POTENTIAL

Scientists have calculated that the potential energy within the average sized person would be equivalent to approximately 150,000 liters of gasoline, enough energy to light up a small town.

Dr. Hans Neiper, M.D.

Dr. Michael A. Schmidt, the author of *Tired of Being Tired: Overcoming Chronic Fatigue and Low Energy*, states that he has seen a significant number of patients regain lost vigor and vim by changing how they live, eat, behave and view life. To fully utilize the innate energy potential Dr. Neiper describes requires some planning. The mistake many health professionals and individual patients make, according to Dr. Schmidt, is becoming preoccupied with the notion that one's loss of energy is due to a single cause. This same sentiment is expressed by Dr. Jacob Teitelbaum, M.D., a board certified medical internist and expert in the treatment of chronic fatigue, fibromyalgia and musculoskeletal pain. In his book, *From Fatigued to Fantastic*, Dr. Teitelbaum cites the fact that chronic fatigue is a direct result of multiple causes, some occurring simultaneously. To regain your lost vitality, vim and vigor, any approach which does not take into consideration the systemic nature of this malady will not eliminate the real underlying causes.

You need to develop a comprehensive plan which will allow you to take a look at all the possible "energy drainers" that perpetuate themselves in your everyday existence. This you have just done with the completion of your individual energy-fatigue profile. It is important now, however, that you begin to formulate an "action plan" that will allow you to eliminate or better manage the problem areas that exist. To get started, please go back and review all the areas of your profile. At first glance, it may seem a bit overwhelming. This, however, is the first step to removing the obstacles that are preventing you from realizing your full energy potential.

Here are some related questions. I hope to answer:

- Just what is an action plan?
- How do I start setting one up?
- How do I set up goals, and should they be long- or short-term?
- Who should be responsible for follow-through once a plan is established?
- Is this plan permanent or can it be altered?
- Can I get others involved with my action plan?
- How often should I evaluate its effectiveness?
- How will I monitor my progress?

In this chapter we shall focus our attention on self-management and our inherent ability to control the illusive entity known as energy.

Developing a Plan of Action

Before setting up a plan of action, it is essential to the success of your program that you keep a few things in mind.

1. For your plan to be effective, it must be fully developed by you.
2. Monitoring and making the necessary adjustments to your plan also has to be done by you.
3. You are the main decision maker who controls all facets of your individual energy — fatigue profile.

4. You need to empower yourself and organize the factors that will produce positive results for you.
5. Have patience with yourself and your outcomes. Give yourself time to reach your goals.
6. Know your physical skill levels but seek ways to expand your abilities.
7. No plan is written in stone — make adjustments and changes when necessary.
8. Seek the help you need to attain your goals.
9. Use the buddy system, get a spouse involved with your program or surround yourself with others whose goals or shared values are similar to yours.
10. Have fun, develop your plan around activities you enjoy and in which have an interest.

Setting Up Your Plan

Steven Silbiger, the author of *The Ten Day* M.B.A. maintains that there are six important steps in developing an action plan. Those steps are:

1. Set specific goals;
2. Define activities, resources needed, responsibilities;
3. Set a timetable for action;
4. Forecast outcomes, develop alternative plans;
5. Formulate a detailed plan of action in time sequence;
6. Implement, supervise execution, and evaluate based on goals in Step One.

Let's briefly review each one of these steps

Step One: Set specific goals

By setting specific goals you will be able to evaluate your efforts and make adjustments as needed.

Step Two: Define activities, resources needed, responsibilities

Once you have established what your goals are, you can then decide on just how you will attain them, what help you need and individual responsibilities.

Step Three: Set a timetable for action

By establishing a timetable this will allow you to set up short-term, mid-term and long-term goals. Do not, however, set up goals that are unrealistic.

Step Four: Forecast outcomes, develop alternative plans

What do you want to happen? Be specific and work toward your expected outcome. Be flexible, make necessary adjustments, as warranted.

Step Five: Formulate a detailed plan of action in time sequence

Here you want to ensure that there are no long gaps in your accomplishments. Be ready to move forward. Establish a time frame for moving into the next phase of your action plan.

Step Six: Implement, supervise execution, and evaluate based on goals in Step One

How are you doing? Does your plan need to be adjusted? Are your time frames and goals realistic? Do you need professional assistance? Are you motivated? Is your plan too rigid? Are you having fun?

Moving Toward the Probable

As you begin to implement your new action plan, you must keep in mind that you are creating an environment for life-long results. Establishing goals that are not realistic will only cause more frustration and fatigue. You should begin setting goals with small timeframes and eventually expand them as you progress forward. If one of your goals is to reassess your skills, your job, or a personal relationship, then do it! If you must find and incorporate a nutritionist into your plan, then do it!

Jeffrey Davison, author of *Blow Your Own Horn*, asserts that he sets goals before dinner, and even on planes. He claims that he is forever setting goals, most of which he discards later, but that's okay. Davison maintains that the process of goal-setting involves much over-reaching initially, followed by a sifting through to find the realistic, attainable gems.

Whatever your goals are:
1. Set realistic goals
2. Be specific

3. Set several related goals
4. Breakdown long-term goals into several short-term goals
5. Enjoy your accomplishments and reward yourself appropriately

In the next section of this chapter you will find a few examples of how to set up a management model with goals, projected outcomes, and other pertinent information.

The power is in your hands, the time for change is now! You are not perfect and you are bound to make mistakes as you formulate and re-assess your action plan, but as you do:

Let no feeling of discouragement prey upon you, and in the end you are sure to succeed.

Abraham Lincoln

A Few Energy Promoting Action Plans

Developing a vision of how you want to be can aid change efforts too. Individuals who are best at producing personal change focus on reducing the discrepancy between where they are now and where they would like to be in the future.

Dr. Murray M. Dalziel, Ph.D.
Dr. Steven C. Schoonover, M.D.
Authors of *Changing Ways*

Preparing For Success

Preparing for success is the first step toward achieving it. However, before formulating an individual action plan it is important to understand that what you are really doing is creating "self-directed" change. To do that, creating and maintaining a positive attitude will help you as you initiate and implement your plan of action. To ensure success, become aware of self-defeating thoughts and habits. Be ready to handle setbacks and changes in your life. Staying focused toward cultivating and managing your energy potential will help you stay on track. First and foremost, begin to break possible negative chains of thought and replace them with positive ones. For example, review the negative thoughts below:

- I don't have the will power
- I'm too old to start making changes now
- I like the way fatty foods taste
- It's useless to try
- I can't function without my morning coffee

Now review the positive 'I can do' self-directed messages that follow:

- I can control my dietary choices
- It's never too late to change unhealthy eating habits
- I will feel more energetic
- I have time, this change doesn't need to occur all at once
- Food is not my only source of pleasure
- I will try herbal teas
- I will find a professional who can assist me with my choices
- I can do this, and I will not wait until tomorrow to start
- My overall health will improve

By developing a positive attitude, the 'how to' will develop as well as the motivation to proceed. Additionally, removing negative connotations will also help you combat stress and general fatigue. There is mounting evidence that your emotions play a critical role in modulating your "stress energy capacity".

Accepting Responsibility

Accept the responsibility for the management of your energy potential by becoming a proactive enforcer of your individual energy plan.

Think Big! Believe you can succeed in increasing your energy and you will. David Schwartz, author of *The Magic of Thinking Big*, states "There is nothing magical or mystical about the power of belief." He maintains that belief works this way:

Belief, the "I'm positive I can" attitude, generates the power, the skill, and energy needed to do. When you believe "I can do it", the "how to do it" develops.

Formulate your plan, implement it and look beyond energy at all the things you could and would like to be doing. Stretch your vision. See what can be done, not just what it is. Make the necessary changes and in the end, a new, more energetic you will emerge.

What To Do

Now that you have a clear picture of where you are and where you want to be, it is time to act. To get started, you should do the following:

- Have appropriate medical tests to rule out the possibility of underlying disease state.
- Use your energy-fatigue profile as your guide in setting up your goals and to identify the areas that need your immediate attention.
- Start preparing your action plan.
- Contact an alternative health professional that deals directly with "energy medicine" and its application for help
- Begin taking a good look at your present dietary regimen and make the necessary adjustments.
- Begin laying out an initial supplement plan to augment your current dietary regimen.
- Set up some daily detox routines.
- Set up guidelines to assess how well your plan is going.
- Have fun and be patient with yourself.

A Simple Plan

As paraphrased by the late Nobel Prize winning chemist Linus Pauling:

No one knows the state of health or energy of a person better than the person himself or herself. It is important to think about one's health and energy and find ways to improve it.

One Hundred And Ninety Ways
To Naturally Improve Your Energy Levels

- **Goal:** To establish some new daily, weekly, or monthly natural protocols that will keep you vibrant, focused, and well-energized.
- **Activity:** By trial and error, based on established protocols, establish routines that are most beneficial.
- **Action Time Table:** Exercise is to be repeated, with new listings and additions once every 3 months.
- **Desired Outcome:** Improvement and daily maintenance of inborn energy potential.
- **Time Sequence:** Interchange, substitute, and make adjustments every two weeks as needed.
- **Consistency of Activity:** Repeat exercise every three months or as changes in lifestyle or events dictate.

One Hundred And Ninety Ways
To Naturally Improve Your Energy Levels

1. Reduce Saturated Fat Intake
2. Limit or Eliminate use of alcoholic beverages
3. Eat more complex carbohydrates
4. Make protein your last snack of the night.
5. Don't overeat
6. Consume 5 to 6 mini-meals
7. Don't skip meals
8. Drink 6 to 8 glasses of clean fresh water daily
9. Begin to use all organic foods
10. Bake rather than fry your foods
11. Eliminate fried foods
12. Reduce intake of processed foods
13. Eliminate or reduce sugar, salt and highly seasoned foods.
14. Consider becoming a vegetarian
15. Don't eat when stressed
16. Eat 5 to 6 servings of fresh vegetables daily
17. Reduce coffee intake, drink herb teas
18. Drink 4 cups of green tea daily

19. Eliminate sugary snacks
20. Make lunch your largest meal of the day
21. Consume 5 to 6 servings of fresh or raw fruit daily.
22. Incorporate various soy products into dietary regimen
23. Eat a variety of foods
24. Replace milk with soy, rice or almond milk.
25. Know your correct calorie ratios
26. Eat your salad last
27. Don't gauge thirst by body's thirst signal—drink!
28. Spike your morning juice with a teaspoon of ginger.
29. Drink one or two vials of ginseng in between meals.
30. Keep fresh, fruit in your desk at work.
31. Drink organic fruit juices
32. Add a teaspoon of lecithin and one teaspoon of wheat germ to your evening beverage.
33. Bring your intake of fiber up to 25-50 grams per day
34. Limit your intake of cakes, pies, candies, and pastries.
35. Have a nutritious mid-morning snack.
36. Exchange ice cream for yogurt
37. Add 1 to 2 teaspoons of sunflower seeds to your yogurt
38. Use soybeans instead of peanuts
39. Consume a protein sports bar in between meals.
40. Switch to low fat milk
41. Use soy milk instead of cream in your coffee.
42. Eat generous helpings of oatmeal.
43. Try low-fat ricotta instead of cream cheese or butter.
44. Try lean ham instead of bacon or sausage.
45. Snack on rice cakes
46. Eat at least 2 hours before a scheduled activity.
47. Eat protein and avoid carbohydrates before a business presentation.
48. Gradually make changes and substitutions to your diet. Do not abruptly discontinue normal food patterns.
49. Switch to soy burgers, or chicken burgers, etc.

50. Eat natural low-calorie snacks
51. Have a fruit carbohydrate drink after exercising
52. Steam your vegetables
53. Avoid canned fruits and vegetables
54. Consume 6 to 8 servings of chicken weekly (preferably antibiotic free)
55. Eat a healthy snack every 3 to 4 hours.
56. Read your labels — avoid, sucrose, dextrose, sorbitol
57. Cook with olive, canola or safflower oil
58. Supplement diet with flax, evening primrose, fish or borage oils
59. Don't eat on the run.
60. Consume generous portions of beans (navy) blackeye peas, lentils.
61. Eliminate luncheon meats
62. Have turkey, tuna or chicken instead of lunch meat
63. Whole grain rice and breads instead of white bread and rice
64. Learn a new nutritious recipe.
65. Space your carbohydrate intake throughout the day
66. Do not eat a full meal right before retiring for the night.
67. Do not drink large amounts of fluids with your meal.
68. Avoid bacon bits, lard, sour cream and vegetable shortening
69. Use fat-free salad dressings-olive oil and vinegar dressings
70. Take a multi-vitamin mineral formula daily
71. Take CoQ10 daily
72. Take a multiple enzyme formula daily
73. Do not overload the system with iron
74. Supplement your diet with Vit. E
75. Eat enough energy foods
76. Add a teaspoon of "MCT" oil to your afternoon sports drink
77. Take an antioxidant supplement.
78. Don't skip Breakfast
79. Watch your food combinations

80. Have a glass of Green Magma, Algae or Chlorella or wheat grass juice.

81. Avoid highly seasoned food

82. Spike your morning juice with a pinch of garlic

83. Utilize the food pyramid

84. Don't eat and go directly to bed.

85. Know your food sensitivity

86. Have 3 cups of licorice root tea daily

87. Don't eat smoked meat fish or fowl

88. Eat generous portions of raw fruits

89. Add 1 to 2 tablespoons of powdered brewer's yeast to 8 oz. of tomato juice

90. Drink naturally decaffeinated coffee if you must drink coffee

91. Opt for raw nuts (except peanuts) instead of roasted nuts

92. Never add salt to the food you are cooking

93. Make protein your last meal of the day.

94. Drink 2 to 3 glasses of vegetable juice daily

95. Start your breakfast high in protein, low in fat with moderate carbohydrates

96. Add a tablespoon of flaxseed oil to your yogurt

97. Do not eat carbohydrates before bedtime

98 Consider using carnitine as a nutritional supplement to speed up metabolism

99. If you are a female are you getting enough iron?

100. Have a choline cocktail at happy hour (mix in non-alcoholic beverage)

101. Eat plenty of grapefruit and lemons

102. Add 1 to 2 tablespoons of barley grass to 8oz of herb tea

103. Recharge your adrenal glands with pantothenic acid (Vit. B5)

104. When building muscle you need at least 3500 calories to produce one pound of muscle

105. Eat right for your metabolic type

106. Replace salsa for most sugar-laden ketchups

107. Avoid palm and cotton-seed oils

108. Take 1000 to 1500 mg. of calcium daily

109. Cycle your calorie intake so that the body will not adapt and slow down metabolic processes.

110. Do not restrict your calorie intake or go on crash diets.

111. Do not totally eliminate fat from you diet.

112. Make sure meats you consume are lean cut

113. Learn how to use the food exchange system.

114. Spike your evening glass of herb tea with spirulina

115. Take one teaspoon of flax seed oil daily.

116. Walk ½ to 2 miles a day

117. Stay active

118. Watch less TV

119. Join a health club

120. Keep your doctor appointments — have yearly or quarterly exams.

121. Know your health indicators (blood pressure, cholesterol etc.)

122. Lose those extra pounds.

123. Don't ignore warning signs of illness.

124. Please don't smoke don't smoke don't smoke.

125. Get some sunshine daily

126. Focus on whole body health

127. Exercise aerobically

128. Go for a swim

129. Soak in the hot tub

130. Take a sauna bath

131. Have your 'Ph' tested

132. Build muscle

133. Park at the far end of the train station

134. Buy and/or use your stationary bike

135. Get more sleep — 7 to 10 hours nightly

136. Keep your colon clean set up monthly detox cycles

137. Consider fasting. Check with your doctor first.

138. Take acidophilus supplements daily.

139. Use 2 week cycles of the herb golden seal once every 3 months.

140. Take an Epson salt bath once every 2 weeks

141. Do a liver cleanse once a quarter

142. Check for yeast infections as a possible cause of your fatigue problems (women)

143. Respect your biological clock
144. Have your thyroid gland checked out
145. Focus on improving immune response
146. After exercising, eat your scheduled meal within 30 to 60 minutes
147. Before a physical event increase your carb intake to 70% for 2 or 3 days before your event.
148. Drink at least 17 ounces of water before a long bike ride
149. Is your job emotionally satisfying?
150. Take a vacation.
151. Take up a new hobby
152. Practice meditation.
153. Know when to say no!
154. Learn how to manage your time
155. Discuss emotional concerns with family and friends
156. Organize your life
157. Develop some goals, don't haphazardly approach projects
158. Pamper yourself
159. Plan for success
160. Learn how to anticipate situations
161. Work smarter, not harder
162. Know your personality type
163. Measure success one day at a time
164. Avoid unnecessary crisis management of life's highs and lows
165. Do it now! Do not procrastinate
166. Take an extra 50 to 100 mg of B-complex vitamins when stressed out.
167. Try the herb Kava or St. Johns Wort to reduce stress and anxiety.
168. Learn the attributes of aromatherapy (the art of scents and fragrances) to reduce stress
169. Do some gardening
170. Schedule a massage
171. Establish routines
172. Plan for change
173. Express yourself
174. Learn to delegate
175. Ask for help
176. Sing a song to someone.
177. Go see a movie
178. Visit a relative
179. Think Positive
180. Learn a new skill
181. Relax, relax, relax

182. Focus on adrenal function with use of adaptogenic supplements

183. Focus beyond the problem, break each problem into small pieces, then solve each piece individually.

184. Learn to play a musical instrument.

185. Paint a picture.

186. Write a poem.

187. Make time for yourself.

188. Write down and define the right situation for you!

189. Avoid self-defeating and negative talk

190. Learn to discuss sexual needs with your partner.

Tracking Energy Action Plan

- Goal: To determine current peaks and valleys of energy and to correlate them with times of the day and night
- Activity: Recording times via tracking chart
- Action Time Table: Exercise to be done for 30 days
- Desired Outcome: Being able to pinpoint possible stressor
- Time Sequence: Tracking to be done every two hours upon rising in the morning until 12:00 a.m.
- Consistency of Activity: Repeat exercise as changes in lifestyle or events dictate

Energy Tracking Chart

	Sun	Mon	Tue	Wed	Thur	Fri	Sat
Time	Time/Score	Time/Score	Time/Score	Time/Score	Time/Score	Time/Score	Time/Score
8:00 AM							
10:00 AM							
12 Noon							
2:00 AM							
4:00 PM							
6:00 PM							
8:00 PM							
10:00 PM							
12:00 AM							

Scoring
0 = Extremely Tired
1 = Low Levels of Energy
2 = Stable Energy Patterns
3 = High Levels of Energy
4 = Very Vibrant

Note: At the end of each week take the times of the day or night you scored the best. From here you can determine what is causing the lower scores at certain time intervals.

Conclusions

Your Energy Plan for Life

It is a professionally based belief that two words from this day forward will become paramount; they are "manage" and "continued experimentation". Your short term immediate goals should focus on becoming an effective manager of your "Individual Action Plan". Peter Drucker, one of the most prolific management theorists, stated that, *"management always has to consider both the present and the future; both the short run and the long run."* According to Drucker, a management problem is not solved if immediate profits endanger the long-range health, perhaps even the survival of a company. As you move forward, remember you are cultivating for life-long results. Start slowly as you formulate your plan. More importantly, become a proactive manager of your action plan.

The second phrase, "continued experimentation", will be the single most important motivational factor that you will encounter. New foods, new studies, new supplements, exercises, new information, improvements in your physical skill level, and most importantly, your management ability, are all factors that will have a profound effect on your future energy levels.

As you begin to move beyond the rudiments of our journey, continue to find ways to master the eight basic principles of energy management cited below:

- Take control of all of the variables found within your Individual Energy-Fatigue Profile and make the necessary adjustments to them as needed!

- Accept the total responsibility for the management of your energy potential by becoming a proactive enforcer of your individual energy building action plan!
- Cultivate and maintain a strong immune response. Without it you cannot compete in the game of life!
- *Become your own personal nutritionist.* Learn as much as you can. Consuming the right fuel (food) at the right time will invigorate your system and switch your energy levels from neutral to turbo-drive!
- Use a synergistic approach to boost your energy levels by supplementing your nutritional program with vitamins, minerals, antioxidants and other accessory supplements!
- Become an expert in stress management. Stress, as we have learned, can have a profound effect on your energy levels as well as your emotional and psychological well-being!
- Keep moving. Become an activist. Research clearly shows that those of us who remain active suffer less from the negative aspects of today's degenerative diseases, have more energy and maintain a healthy, positive attitude about ourselves!

Beyond Energy

You need to look beyond your present energy level (or lack of it) as simply the way it is. You have, right now, the ability and knowledge to reach and enjoy your full metabolic energy potential.

The final lever in this process, however, is you! You must now begin to put your new base of knowledge into action! As stated by Dr. A. Bandura, Ph.D. of Stanford University:

> Your belief in yourself can influence how much effort you make to change, whether you persevere or give up in the face of obstacles, and how much stress you experience while you're changing your life. Don't wait for others to make decisions for you. Take charge of your lifestyle and your environment, and change those influences that derail your progress.

For additional help, please see Appendix E, found in the rear of this book, "Getting the Help You Need".

EPILOGUE

When energy is viewed from a biological standpoint it quickly becomes evident that energy is not an elusive entity, but a interminable, pulsating, dynamic force which is always present. When energy is examined in this context, it also becomes evident that we, the earth, flowers, plants, animals, and what is known as the cosmos, are all intertwined with the extraordinary process of energy production and exchange. And it is evident that this process is a perfectly boundless process.

When human bioenergetics is viewed from a physiological standpoint, it immediately becomes apparent that the human body is nothing more than a river of pure energy. You are essentially an energy transformation plant, a venerable holding station with an unlimited and an inexhaustible potential to convert, transform, and utilize a variety of biological sources of energy.

In essence, energy, nature's sources of energy, and human physiology are one in the same. When viewed from this context, one can see why scientists contend that you have an unlimited energy potential.

Furthermore, when human energetics is viewed from a biological standpoint, it becomes evident that fatigue or lack of energy is a direct result in the interruption of nature's intended metabolic energy producing pathways, whether self, genetically, or environmentally imposed.

Each one of us is born with the capability to produce, enjoy, and realize nature's intended energy potential for life. The key in attaining and sustaining a high level of energy over one's lifetime is clearly embodied in Dr. Andrew Weil's comment, which was

Health and Energy Ought to Flow from the Way We Live!

In the absence of any genetic defects you have the ability to produce all the energy you will ever need. Please begin incorporating the programs outlined here in *Energy For Life*. You and you alone control your energy potential. You are the key! Good luck and, as always, **Good Health To You!**

Appendices

Appendix A

ENERGY TO GO

Some Energy Recipes

In addition to trying the supplements cited in this book you may want to consider the following recipes for a quick energy boost. The ingredients are inexpensive, easy to make, and they are not artificial stimulants:

The Young Vigor Tonic
1 tablespoon lecithin powder or granules mixed into a glass of organic tomato juice
Add one tablespoon brewer's yeast
Stir vigorously
Drink one glass before each meal and one at bedtime

The Energy Elixir
(for the habitual coffee-drinker)
2 tablespoons of powdered brewer's yeast
½ cup skimmed milk
½ cup soy milk
1 tablespoon organic raw honey

Yeast Cocktail
(for internal revitalization)
> Mix four tablespoons of powdered brewer's yeast in fresh fruit
> or vegetable juice
> Season with honey to your taste
> Drink one glass, at least 3-4 times a day

Nature Sweet Raw Juice
(as a pick me up)
> Mix ½ cup of grape juice with ½ cup of apple juice
> Two mashed bananas
> Blend together
> Drink one glass before meals or in between meals
> instead of high calorie, sugar-laden snacks.
> Note: Please use fresh raw juices. Juices in their
> concentrated form are not "raw"

The Casanova Cocktail
(to increase sexual prowess)
> ½ teaspoon cinnamon powder
> ½ cup slightly steamed apple juice
> ½ cup grapefruit juice
> Mix all ingredients vigorously and drink slowly

Heart-Health Revitalizer
> ½ cup organic tomato juice, preferably not from concentrate
> 1 tablespoon brewer's yeast powder
> ½ cup organic citrus juice, preferably fresh squeezed
> 6 tablespoons of cold-pressed wheat germ oil
> Mix in blender or stir vigorously. Drink one glass during early
> morning, one a few hours after lunch, and one a few hours
> after dinner.

Raw Juice Heart Tranquilizer

10 tablespoons of wheat germ oil
½ cup fresh carrot juice
½ cup fresh lettuce juice
1 tablespoon fresh lemon juice
Stir vigorously and drink daily

For Anemia and Tired Blood

Juice 8 carrots, two beets and six
ounces of celery in a food blender
or juicer. Drink daily.

Appendix B

ANTI-IMMUNITY AND PRO-IMMUNITY FOODS

Anti-Immunity Foods

The foods in this table should be avoided to minimize your risk of diet-induced cancer and to promote maximum immune readiness.

Food Category	Foods to Avoid
Beverages	Alcohol; cocoa; coffee; flavored and colored beverages; canned and pasterized juices; artificial fruit drinks; all artificially sweetened drinks; non-dairy creamers.
Dairy Products	All processed and imitation butter, ice cream, and toppings; all orange and pasteurized cheeses.
Eggs	Fried.
Fish	Deep-fried.
Fruit	Canned, sweetened.
Grains	White flour products; hull-less grains and seed (e.g. pasta, crackers, snack foods, white rice, prepared or cold cereals, cooked seeds).
Meats	All red meat products should be reduced and eventually eliminated.
Nuts	Roasted and/or salted, especially peanuts.
Oils	Shortening; refined fats and oils (unsaturated as well as saturated); hydrogenated margarine.
Seasonings	Pepper; excessive use of hot spices.
Soups	Canned and creamed (thickened); commercial bouillon-fat stock
Sweets	Refined sugars (white, brown, turbinado); chocolate; candy; syrups; all artificial sweets.
Vegetables	Canned; deep-fried potatoes in any form; corn chips.

Additional recommendations: Avoid foods that have been sprayed with insecticides, food additives (especially monosodium glutamate [MSG], and others ending in "-ate"), and foods with artificial colors, flavors and preservatives.

Pro-Immunity Foods

The foods in this table are recommended for promoting optimal immunity and for minimizing your risk of diet-induced cancer.

Food Category	Recommended Foods
Beverages	Herb teas (e.g. Maitake, chamomile, mint, papaya——no caffeine); fresh fruit and vegetable juices, soy, rice, multi-grain and almond milk
Dairy Products	Raw milk, yogurt, butter, buttermilk, nonfat cottage cheese, uncolored unprocessed cheese.
Eggs	Poached or soft-boiled.
Fish	Fresh white-fleshed, broiled or baked.
Fruit	All dried (unsulfured), stewed, fresh, and frozen (unsweetened).
Grains	Whole grain cereals, bread, muffins (e.g. rye, oats, wheat, bran, buckwheat, millet); cream of wheat, brown rice.
Meats	Gradually reduce.
Nuts and Seeds	All fresh, raw, or dry roasted (unsalted). Also whole seeds (sesame, pumpkin, sunflower, flaxseed).
Oils	Cold-pressed oils——olive; peanut.
Seasonings	Herbs——garlic, onion, rosemary, parsley, marjoram.
Soups	Any made from scratch (e.g., salt-free vegetable, chicken, barley, millet, brown rice).
Sprouts	Especially wheat, pea, lentil, mung, and alfalfa.
Sweets	Pure, unfiltered honey, unsulfured molasses, pure maple syrup (in limited amounts only) and stevia.
Vegetables	All raw, steamed, and lightly sauteed, fresh or frozen; potatoes, baked or boiled.

Appendix C

WHAT IS YOUR ANTIOXIDANT PROFILE

Answer each of the following questions. Then calculate your score by checking the answers at the end of this Quiz. Add them up, and determine your Antioxidant Profile.

1. How many servings of yellow-orange fruits and leafy green or yellow-orange vegetables do you have daily?
   a. 2 to 4 half-cup or equivalent size servings
   b. 5 to 9 half-cup or equivalent size servings
   c. less than 2 half-cup servings

2. Are the vegetables that you eat mostly fried, baked, boiled, steamed or raw?
   a. fried   d. steamed
   b. baked   e. raw
   c. boiled

3. Do you use "cold-pressed" vegetable oil?
   a. yes   b. no

4. How often do you travel by airplane?
   a. more than 6 times a month
   b. about 2 to 4 times a month
   c. less than once a month

179

5. How much time do you spend outdoors?
   a. more than 20 hours a week
   b. about 5 to 20 hours a weak
   c. less than 5 hours a week

6. Do you smoke cigarettes?
   a. yes   b. no

7. Do you have more than one or two alcoholic beverages a day?
   a. yes   b. no

8. How close do you live to a city or an industrial manufacturing complex?
   a. live in city or near an industrial manufacturing complex
   b. live in suburbs of city or several miles away from an industrial manufacturing complex
   c. live in rural area, far from a city or an industrial manufacturing complex

9. How often do you exercise?
   a. 3 or 4 times a week, for about 30 minutes each session
   b. more than 5 times a week, each session lasting more than 30 minutes
   c. less than 2 times a week

10. Are you taking an antioxidant formula to supplement your diet?
   a. yes   b. no

Your Score

Below are the answers to the Antioxidant Profile Quiz. Each response is given a numeric value. A value of five is the most positive, and lower values may mean areas that need improvement.

1. a. 2 You are not obtaining protective amounts of antioxidants from fruits and vegetables, leaving cells vulnerable to free radical destruction; eat three to five more servings a day.

b. 5 You're getting valuable antioxidants from fruits and vegetables, especially if the vegetables are eaten raw.

c. 0 You're not getting any antioxidants from fruits and vegetables; to help protect cells from free radical damage, eat five to nine servings a day.

2. a. 1 Frying is high in fat and heat destroys some antioxidants.
   b. 3 Baking is healthy, but usually requires the addition of fat, and involves the loss of some antioxidants to heat.
   c. 2 Antioxidants are lost through leaching and heat.
   d. 4 Steaming is a healthy cooking option, but it destroys some antioxidants.
   e. 5 Raw, fresh vegetables supply the most intact antioxidants.

3. a. 5 More vitamin E remains in cold-pressed vegetable oil than in oil processed with heat.
   b. 0 Certain vegetable oils are good sources of polyunsaturated fats, which are associated with helping to lower cholesterol levels. However, heat processing destroys vitamin E, increasing your need for this vitamin.

4. a. 1 Excessive exposure to sunlight and ambient radiation may increase free radical activity, possibly increasing the need for protective antioxidants.
   b. 2 Moderate exposure to sunlight and ambient radiation may have an effect on free radical activity, possibly increasing the need for protective antioxidants.
   c. 5 Limited outdoor activity decreases your exposure to the harmful effects of the sun.

5. a. 0 Research indicates that airline passengers may be exposed to relatively high levels of radiation; the more one flies, the greater the exposure. Studies show that radiation may be associated with increased free radical activity, increasing the need for cell-protecting antioxidants.

b. 3 Moderate air travel exposes passengers to greater levels of radiation than if traveling by ground transportation. Even this amount of radiation exposure affects free radical activity, increasing the need for antioxidants.

c. 5 Limited air travel lessens your exposure to elevated radiation levels associated with airline flights; therefore, your requirement for antioxidants is not affected by this activity.

6. a. 0 Smoking may greatly increase the need for protective antioxidants. Vitamins E and C work synergistically to protect lung cells from free radical activity caused by smoking.

 b. 5 Yet another good reason not to smoke, as research shows that it may increase the need for antioxidants.

7. a. 0 High intakes of alcohol may greatly increase the need for all the antioxidants, particulary selenium. Moreover, all nutrients may be affected by high alcohol intake.

 b. 5 Moderate to no intake of alcohol does not affect your requirement for antioxidants.

8. a. 2 Air pollution may increase your need for antioxidants.

 b. 3 You may be exposed to some of the air pollution from a nearby city or industrial manufacturing plant.

 c. 5 Even when living in a pollution-free environment, normal body metabolism requires antioxidants to battle free radicals.

9. a. 4 Although exercise increases your need for antioxidants, experts recommend a moderate exercise program to maintain good health. Adding a vitamin and mineral supplement insures protective amounts of antioxidants, particularly during physical stress.

 b. 3 Excessive exercise increases your need for many nutrients, including antioxidants.

 c. 5 Exercise increases the need for antioxidants. However, by not exercising regularly, you are likely to have more body fat, be overweight, and have an increased risk of associated diseases.

10. a. 5 You are assured of getting the protective amounts of antioxidants.
    b. 0 You may not be getting protective amounts of antioxidants every day.

Your Antioxidant Profile

45 to 50: Excellent. You know how to live a healthy lifestyle and protect your cells with a diet rich in antioxidants — the nutrients that research shows may help to protect your body's cells from the ravaging effects of free radicals.

35 to 44: You're on the right track, but you may need to strengthen your cell-protecting antioxidant profile. Review the questions, and determine which areas need greater attention.

Less than 35: You need help! Review this outline, and determine which areas need work. By improving your antioxidant profile, you will help prevent the destructive damage of natural body processes on cells.

YOUR INDIVIDUAL FATIGUE PROFILE

The Brain Longevity Stress Impact Index

Event	Stressor Rating	Personal Perception Multiplier (1-10)	Score
Death of your Child	100	_____	_____
Death of your Spouse	99	_____	_____
Life-threatening illness	95	_____	_____
Prison term	80	_____	_____
Divorce	78	_____	_____
Marital separation	68	_____	_____
Death of a parent or sibling	68	_____	_____
Fired from your job	65	_____	_____
Pregnancy	60	_____	_____
Hospitalization for serious illness	58	_____	_____
Marriage	57	_____	_____
Foreclosure on mortgage	57	_____	_____
Serious illness in the family	55	_____	_____
Birth of a child	50	_____	_____
Demotion at work	50	_____	_____

Lawsuit against you	50	_____	_____
Retirement	49	_____	_____
Sexual problems	45	_____	_____
Laid off from work	43	_____	_____
Problems with boss	40	_____	_____
Major business change	40	_____	_____
Major change in finance	39	_____	_____
Move to new town	38	_____	_____
Death of a close friend	38	_____	_____
Change of career	38	_____	_____
Change in frequency of arguments with spouse of significant other	35	_____	_____
Change in sleep habits	31	_____	_____
Problems with co-workers	30	_____	_____
Assuming a mortgage of over 25 percent of net earnings	29	_____	_____
Birth of first grandchild	28	_____	_____
Children leaving home	27	_____	_____
Problems with extended family	25	_____	_____
Significant life style change	24	_____	_____
Illness of more than one week duration	23	_____	_____
Promotion at work	23	_____	_____
Change in political or religious beliefs	20	_____	_____
Assuming a mortgage of over 20 percent of net earning	18	_____	_____
Change in social life	17	_____	_____
Change in diet	15	_____	_____
Vacation	10	_____	_____
Minor legal problem	10	_____	_____

Total Score_____

If the sum of your multiplied scores (your total score) is less than 500, you are leading a relatively stress-free life. If it is 500 to 1,000, you have a low-stress life. If it is 1,000 to 2,000, you have a life of moderate stress and should work hard to minimize your response to your stressors. If your score is 2,000 to 3,000, you have high-stress life, one that is almost certainly creating short term cognitive dysfunction and that may eventually contribute to age-associated cognitive decline. if your score is higher than 3,000, you are in the danger zone, your stress levels are far too high and are a serious threat to your physical health, emotional well-being, cognitive function and brain longevity. If you had a high total score on the Stress Impact Index, it means that you are habitually experiencing the "stress response." It is the stress response that physically endangers you.

Appendix E

GETTING THE HELP
YOU NEED

**The Holistic Health
Energy Directory**

Organizations

Center for Medical Consumers
237 Thompson St.
New York, NY 10012
212-674-7105

National Health Information
Clearing House
P.O. Box 1133
Washington, DC 20013

The Chronic Fatigue and Immune
Dysfunction Syndrome Association
of America
P.O. Box 220398
Charlotte, NC 28222-0398
800-442-3437

American Association for Chronic
Fatigue Syndrome
P.O. Box 895
Olney, MD 20830

American Association of Alternative
Healers
P.O. Box 10026
Sedona, AZ 86336
520-345-8622

American Association of Naturopathic
Physicians
2366 E. Lake Ave. East Suite 322
Seattle, WA 98102
206-298-0126

American Association of Nutritional
Consultants
810 S. Buffalo St.
Warsaw, IN 46580
888-228-AANC

American Academy of Allergy and
immunology
611 W. Wells St.
Milwaukee, WI 53202
414-272-6071

National Organization for Seasonal
Affective Disorder
P.O. Box 40133
Washington, D.C. 20016

American Preventive Medical
Association
459 Walker Rd.
Great Falls, VA 22066
703-759-0662

Web Sites & Hotlines

Web Sites

National Library of Medicine (Medline)
http://www.nim.nih.gov

Office of Inspector General -U.S. Department of Health and Human Services
http://www.sba.gov./ignet/internal/hhs.html

Health Gate
http://www.healthgate.com

Natural Medicine Forum (on Compuserve)
GONATMED

Health World Online
http://www.healthy.net

Hotlines

World Research Foundation
818-999-5483

Chronic Fatigue Syndrome Hotline
800-Help-CFS (435-7237)

National Chronic Fatigue Syndrome and Fibromyalgia Association Hotline
Kansas City, Missouri
816-313-2000

Atkins Center for Complimentary Medicine
212-758-2110

The M.D.'s Holistic Health Line
900-Get-Well

Appendix E

Suggested Reading

Atkinson, H., *Women and Fatigue*. G.P. Putnam's and Sons, New York, NY, 1985.

Bennion, L., *Hypoglycemia: Fact or Fad?*. Crown Publishers, New York, NY, 1983.

Berger, S. M., *Forever Young*, William Morrow and Co., Inc., New York, NY, 1989.

Bolles, R., *The Three Boxes of Life and How To Get Out of Them*. Ten Speed Press, Berkley, CA, 1981

Brown, B. B., *Supermind: The Ultimate Energy*, Harper and Row, New York, 1980.

Burns, D., *Feeling Good*. New American Library, New York, 1980.

Carson, R.D., *Taming Your Gremlin: A Guide To Enjoying Yourself*. Harper and Row, New York, NY, 1986.

Chopra, D., *Ageless Body, Timeless Mind*. Harmony Books, New York, NY, 1993.

Diamond, J., *Life Energy*. Vital Health Publishing, Bloomingdale, IL, 1995.

Haas, R., *Eat To Win*. Penguin Books, New York, NY, 1983.

Health For Life, *The Human Fuel Handbook*, Health For Life, Los Angeles, CA, 1988.

Laken, A., *How To Get Control of Your Time and Manage Your Life*. Signet, New York, NY, 1974.

Lamb, L., *Metabolics: Putting Your Food Energy To Work*, Harper and Row, New York, NY, 1974.

Morehouse, L.E., Gross, L., *Total Fitness in Thirty Minutes a Week*. Pocket Books, New York, 1987

Pauling, L., *How To Live Longer and Feel Better*, W.H. Freeman and Co., New York, NY, 1986.

Pearsall, P., *Superimmunity: Master Your Emotions and Improve Your Health*. Fawcett, New York, NY, 1987.

Perry, S., and Dawson, J., *The Secrets Our Body Clocks Reveal*. Rawson Associates, New York, 1988.

Robertson, J., *Peak Performance Living*. Harper/Collins, San Francisco, CA, 1996.

Schuller, R.H., *Tough Times Never Last But Tough People Do!* Bantam Books, New York, NY, 1984.

Sheehy, G., *Passages: Predictable Crises of Adult Life*. Bantam Books, New York, NY, 1977.

Shone, R., *Creative Visualization: How To Use Imagery and Imagination for Self Improvement*. Thorsons, Rochester, VT, 1984.

Vierk, E., *Health Smart, Your Personal Plan to Living Longer and Healthier*. Prentice Hall, Englewood Cliffs, NJ, 1995.

Wade, C., *Health Secrets for the Orient*. Parker Publishing Co., West Nyack, NY, 1973.

Wade, C., *Health Tonics, Elixirs and Potions for the Look and Feel of Youth*. Parker Publishing Co., West Nyack, NY, 1971.

Watson, D.L., Roland, G.T., *Self-Directed Behavior: Self-Modification for Personal Adjustment*. Brooks-Cole Publishers, Monterey, CA, 1985.

References

Chapter One

Asimov, I.; *The Chemicals of Life*, New American Library, New York, NY, 1954.

Brady, J.E., and Holum, J.R.; *Fundamentals of Chemistry*, John Wiley and Sons, New York, NY, 1984.

Bieler, H.C.; *Food Is Your Best Medicine*, Random House, New York, NY, 1968.

Carlson, L.D., and Hsieh, A.C.L.; *Control of Energy Exchange*, The MacMillan Co., New York, NY, 1970.

Cichoke, A.J.; *Boost Your Energy*, The Energy Times, Long Beach, CA, September/October 1995, P. 22-28 & 6.

Curtis, H.; *Biology*; 4th Ed., Worth Publishers, Inc. 1983.

Hoch, Folo; *Energy Transformation in Mammals*; Regulatory Mechanisms, W.B. Saunders, Philadelphia, PA, 1971.

Kervran, L.; *Biological Transmutations*, Swan Publishing, Binghamton, NY, 1972.

Lamb, L.E.; *Metabolics: Putting Your Food Energy to Work*, Harper and Row, New York, NY, 1974.

Mathews, A.P.; *Physiological Chemistry*, William Wood and Company, New York, NY, 1931.

Starr, C., Taggart; *Biology: The Unity and Diversity of Life*, 4th Ed., Wadsworth Publishing Co., Belmont, CA, 1987.

Williams, S.R.; *Essentials of Nutrition and Diet Therapy*, C.V. Musby Philadelphia, PA, 1978.

Chapter 2

Asimov, I.; *The Chemicals of Life*, The New American Library, New York, NY 1954.

Birkmayer, C.D., *NADH; The Energizing Coenzyme*, Menuco, Corporation, New York NY, 1996.

Buskirk, 'ER' Mendez, J.; Energy: Calorie Requirements (Laboratory For Human Performance Research, Intercollege Research Programs, Penn State University, University Park, PA) Found in Human Nutrition: A comprehensive Treatise, Edited by Roslyn B. Alfm - Slater and David Kritchevsly, Plenum Press, New York, NY, 1980.

Chopra, D., *Boundless Energy*, Harmony Books, New York, NY, 1995.

Fargo, F., Lagnado, J.J., *Life In Action*, Vintage Books, New York, NY, 1975.

Garrison, R, and Somer, E., *The Nutrition Desk Reference*, New Cannan, CT, 1995 (Keats Publishing).

Greenhaff, Polo, et al.; "Influence of Oral Creatine Supplementation on Muscle Phosphocreatine Resynthesis Following Intense Contraction in Man," *Journal of Applied Physiology* v, 467 (1993): 7 5.

Herrington,, D.E., *How to Read Schematic Diagrams*, Howard W. Sams, and Co./NC, Indianapolis, IN, 1967.

King, B.C., Showers, M.J., *Human Anatomy and Physiology*, W.B. Saunders, Philadelphia, PA, 1969.

Krebs, E.C., Beavo, J.A.; *Phosphorylation — Dephosphorylation of Enzymes*, Annual Rev. Biochemistry 48: 923, 1979.

Lamb, L.E. Metabolics, *Putting Your Food Energy To Work*, Harper and Row, New York, NY., 1974.

Mathews, AP., *Physiological Chemistry*, William Wood and Co., New York, NY 1931.

Memmler, R.L., Cohen, B.J. and Wood, D.L., *The Human Body in Health and Disease*, Lippencott, Philadelphia, PA, 1996.

Nature's Plus, *The Complete Book on Energy*, Long Beach, CA, 1995.

Neurath, H., "The Versatility of Proteolyfic Enzymes," *Journal of Cell Biochemistry* 32: 35, 1986.

Pearson. D., Shaw, S., *Life Extension*, Warner Books, New York, NY, 1982.

Pfeiffer, J., *The Cell*, Time Life Books, New York, NY, 1972.

Ratcliff J.D., *Your Body and How It Works*, Readers Digest and Delaconke Press, 1975.

Slater, L.C., "The Mechanism of the Conservation of Energy of Biological Oxidafions;" *Eur. Journal of Biology*, 166:489, 1987.

Starr C., Taggert, R; *Biology: The Unity and Diversity of Life*, 4 Ed, Wadsworth Publishing Co., Belmont, CA, 1987.

Webster's Dictionary, Random House, New York, NY, 1980.

Weil, A; *Health and Healing*, Houghton Co., New York, NY, 1995.

Chapter Three

Asimov, I., *The Chemical of Life*, The New American Library, Inc., New York, NY, 1954.

Becker, W., *Energy and The Living Cell: An Introduction to Bioenergetics*, Lippincott Publishers, Philadelphia, PA, 1977.

Cichoke, A.J., "Boost Your Energy", *the Energy Times Magazine*, Long Beach, CA, Sept/Oct, 1995, p. 22-28.

Cichoke, A.J., "Enzymes: Biological Catalysts," *Health Foods Magazine*, PTN Publishing Group, Melville, NY., June, 1994 p.49-50.

Cichoke, A.J., *Enzymes and Enzyme Therapy: How to Jump Start Your Way to Good Health*, Keats Publishing, New Caannan, CT, 1994.

Conway, J.M., *Energy Metabolism, in Diet and Nutrition Source Book, Vol. 15*; Ed., D.R. Harris, Omnigraphics Inc., Detroit, MI, 1996, p. 389-396.

Crayhon, R., "Energy Therapy", *Total Health*, Vol. 20, No 1, St. George, UT, 1998, p. 14-15.

Davis, F., *Living Alive*, Doubleday and Co., Inc., Garden City, NY, 1980.

Farago, P., Lagnado, J., *Life In Action*, Vintage Books, New York, 1973.

Hatfield, T.C., and Zucker, M., "Improving Your Energy Levels Nutritionally", *Weider Health and Fitness*, Woodland Hills, CA, 1990.

Kervran, C.L., *Biological Transmutations*, Swan House Publishing Co., Binghamton, NY, 1972.

King, B.G., and Showers, M.J., *Human Anatomy and Physiology*, 6th ED., W.B. Saunders Co., Philadelphia, PA, 1969.

Mathews, A.P., *Physiological Chemistry*, William Wood and Co. 5th ED., 1931.

Montgomery, R., Conway, T.W., Spector, A.A., *Biochemistry: A Case-Oriented Approach*, C.V. Mosby, Philadelphia, PA, 1990.

Pfeiffer, J., *The Cell*, Time Life Books, New York, NY, 1972.

Starr, C., Taggart, R., *Biology: The Unity and Diversity of Life*, Wadsworth Publishing Co., Belmont, CA, 1987.

Williams, S.R., *Essentials of Nutrition and Diet Therapy*, C.N. Mosby Co., St. Louis, MO, 1978.

Wilson, M., *Energy*, Time-Life Books, New York, NY, 1967.

Chapter Four

Airola, P., *How To Get Well*, Health Plus Publishers, Sherwood, OR, 1989, p.24.

Anderson, H.L., and Heindel, M.B., et.al., "Effect on Nitrogen Balance of Adult Man of Varying Source in Nitrogen Level of Calorie Intake", *Journal of Nutrition*, 1969: 82-90.

Atkins, R.C., *Dr. Atkins Vita-Nutrient Solution*, Simon and Schuster, New York, NY, 1998, p.32.

Berger, S., *How To Be Your Own Nutritionist*, William Morrow and Co., New York, NY, 1987.

Bland, J., *Assess Your Own Nutritional Status*, Keats Publishing, New Canaan, CT, 1982.

Bagardus, C. La Grange, et.al., "Comparison of Carbohydrate-containing and carbohydrate restricted hypocaloric diets in the treatment of obesity", *Journal of Clinical Investigation*, 1981: 68: 399-404.

Bohannon, K., F., "Endocrine responses to sugar ingestion in man", *Journal of the American Dietetic Association*, 1980: (76): 555-560.

Brody, J., *Jane Brody's Nutrition Book*, Bantam Books, New York, N.Y, 1982.

Clark, N., *Nancy Clark's Sports Nutrition Guide Book*; Leisure Press, Champaign, IL, 1990.

Cichoke, A.J., *Enzymes: Biological Catalysts, Health Foods*, PTN Publishing Group, Melville, NY, June, 1994, p.49-50.

Coleman, E., *Eating For Endurance*, Bull Publishing, Palo Alto, CA, 1988.

Conway, J.M., *Energy Metabolism, In Diet and Nutrition Source Book*, (D.R. Harris, ed.) Omingraphics Inc., Detroit, MI, 1996. P 389-396.

Coyle, E.F., and Coggan, A.R., "Effectiveness of Carbohydrate Feeding in Delaying Fatigue during Prolonged Exercise", *Journal of Sports Medicine*, 1984: 446-458.

Crayhon, R., *Robert Crayhon's Nutrition Made Simple*, M. Evans and Co., Inc., New York, NY, 1994.

Dunne, L.T., *Nutrition Almanac*, McGraw Hill, New York, N.Y, 1990.

Fargo, P., Lagnado, J., *Life In Action*, Vintage Books, New York, N.Y, 1973.

Farguhar, J.W., Frank, A., et.al., "Glucose, Insulin, and Triglyceride Responses to High and Low Carbohydrate Diets in Man," *Journal of Clinical Investigation*, 1966; (45): 1648-1656.

FDA Consumer, "Focus on Food Labeling", U.S. Food and Drug Administration, Rockville, MD, May, 1993.

Flatt, J.P., "The Biochemistry of Energy Expenditure.", in Recent Advances in Obesity Research (ed.G. Brady) John Libbey and Co. London, 1978. P. 211-228.

References

Garza, C., Scrimshaw, N.S., and Young, V.R., "Human Protein Requirements: The Effects of Variations in Energy Intake Within the Maintenance Range.", *American Journal of Clinical Nutrition*, Vol. 29, 1976; (29); 280-287.

Gastelu, D., and Hatfield, F., *Dynamic Nutrition for Maximum Performance*, Avery Publishing Group, Garden City Park, N.Y, 1997.

Gittleman, A.L., *Your Body Knows Best*, Pocket Books, New York, NY, 1996.

Gittleman, A.L., *The 40/30/30/ Phenomenon*, Keats Publishing, New Canaan CT, 1997.

Graham, D., "Food Combining The Missing Link to Better Nutrition", *Let's Live*, Los Angeles CA, 10:94:58-60.

Haas, R., *Eat To Succeed*, Rawson Associates, New York, N.Y, 1986.

Haas, R., *Eat To Win*, Penguin Books, New York N.Y, 1983.

Hatfield, F.C., and Zucker, M., "Improving Your Energy Levels Nutritionally", *Weider Health and Fitness*, Woodland Hills, CA, 1990.

Heyer, A.A., *A Beginner's Introduction to Nutrition*, Keats Publishing, New Canaan, CT, 1983.

Horton, E., and Terjung, R., *Exercise, Nutrition, and Energy Metabolism*, Macmillan Publishing Co., New York, NY, 1988.

Karlsson, J., Saltin, B., "Diet, Muscle Glycogen and Endurance Performance", *Journal of Applied Physiology*, 1971; (31): 203-206.

Katahn, M., *One Meal at a Time*, W.W. Norton and Co., New York, 1991.

King, B.G., Showers, M.J., *Human Anatomy and Physiology 6th ed.*, W.B. Saunders, Phila. PA, 1969.

Kleiner, S.M., *Power Eating*, Human Kinetics, Champaign, IL 1998 p.50.

Kromhout, D., "N-3 fatty acids and coronary heart disease: Epidemiology from eskimos to western populations", *Journal of Internal Medicine*, 1989: 225 (731): 47-51.

Landis, R., *Herbal Defense*, Warner Books, New York, NY, 1997.

Lamb, L.E., Metabolics, *Putting Your Food Energy To Work*, Harper and Row, New York, N.Y, 1974.

Lenfant, C., and Ernest, N., Daily Dietary Fat and Total Food — Energy Intakes, Hanes (National Health and Nutrition Examination Survey III, Phase I, 1988-91), *Journal of American Medical Association*, 1994; 217:1309.

Luoma, T.C., *Food Facts For Fit Folks*, Muscle Media Inc., Golden CO, Sept. 1997, p. 91-97.

Marckman, P., and Sandstrom, B., et.al., "Effects of total Fat Content and Fatty Acid Composition in Diet on Factor VII and Blood Lipids. *Artherosclerosis*, 1990: 80 (3) : 227-233.

Mattson, F.H., "A Changing Role for Dietary Monounsaturated Fatty Acids", *Journal of the American Dietetic Association*, 1989; 89 (3): 387-391.

Mattson, K.F., *A Search For Wellness*, Super G. Publishing, Hampton VA, 1990.

McNutt, K., Mcnutt, D., *Nutrition and Food Choices*, Science Research Associates Inc., Chicago, IL, 1978.

Mitchell, J.B., Costill, J.J., et.al., "Effects of Carbohydrate and Science in Sports and Exercise", Vol 20, No. 2, 1998: 110-115.

National Research Council, *Recommended Dietary Allowances*, (10th ed), National Academy Press, Washington, D.C., 1989.

Nature's Plus, *Spiru-Teen Weight Loss Program*, Long Beach CA, 1997.

Pauling, L., *How To Live Longer and Feel Better*, W.H. Freeman and Co., New York, NY, 1986.

Raymond, C., "Be In Balance", *Natural Way Magazine*, Natural Way Publications, Irvington, NY., 10533, March/April 1999, p. 48-51.

Robertson, J., *Peak Performance Living*, Harper Collins San Francisco, CA, 1996.

Saltman, P., Gurnin, J., and Mothner, I., *The California Nutrition Book*, Little Brown and Co., Boston MA, 1987.

Saunders, J., and Ross, H.M., *Hypoglycemia: The Disease Your Doctor Won't Treat*, Pinnacle Books, Windsor Publishing Corp, New York, NY, 1980.

Sears, B. Lawren, B., *Enter The Zone*, Harper and Collins, New York, NY, 1995.

Smith, N.J., *Food For Sport*, Bull Publishing Co., Palo Alto, CA, 1976.

United States Department of Agriculture, "Energy Value of Foods", *Agriculture Handbook No.74.*, 1973.

Somer, E., *Food and Mood*, Henry Holt and Co., New York, NY, 1995.

Stone, N.J., "Diet, Lipids, and Coronary Heart Disease," *Endocrinology and Metabolism Clinics of North America*, 1990; 19 (2): 321-344.

Switzer, J., *New Stacking Special Report*, Next Nutrition, Carlsbad CA, 1996.

Tierra, L., *The Herbs of Life*, The Crossing Press Freedom CA, 1992.

Tietelbaum, J., *From Fatigued To Fantastic!*, Avery Publishing Group, Garden City Park NY, 1996.

Wade, W., *Health Secrets From the Orient*, Parker Publishing, West Nyack, NY, 1973.

Wade, W., *Health Tonics Elixirs and Potions*, Parker Publishing, West Nyack, NY, 1971.

Wolever, T.M., and Jenkins, D.J., A., et.al., "The Glycemic Index: Methodology and Clinical Implications", *American Journal of Clinical Nutrition* 1991; (54): 846-854.

Wolever, T.M., Jenkins, D.J.A., and Collier, C.R., et.al., "Metabolic Response To Test Meals Containing different carbohydrate foods: Relationship between rate of digestion and plasma insulin response", *Nutrition Research*, 1988; (8): 573-581.

References

Wurtman, J.J., *Managing Your Mind and Mood Through Food*, Rawson Associates, New York, NY, 1986.

Young, V.R., "Protein and Amino Acid requirements in Humans", *Scandinavian Journal of Nutrition*, 1992; (36): 47-56.

Zawadzki, K.M., Yaspelkis, B.B., and Ivy, J.L., Carbohydrate-protein Complex increases the rate of Muscle Glycogen Storage after exercise", *Journal of Applied Physiology*, 1992;(72): 1854-1859.

Chapter Five

Antonio, J., *The Amino Files*, Muscle And Fitness, Woodland Hills Ca., 3:98: 163-167.

Bland, J., *Octacosanol, Carnitine, and Other Accessory Nutrients*, Keats Publishing, New Canaan, CT, 1982.

Birkmayer, C.D., *NADH, The Energizing Coenzyme*, Menuco, Co, New York, NY, 1996.

Challem, J., "CoQ10, May Be the 90's Miracle Nutrient", *Let's Live*, Los Angeles, CA, 8:95: 18-22.

Clouatre, D., Brink, W., "Alpha Lipoic Acid For Total Performance", *Let's Live*, Los Angeles, CA, 10:97: 65-67.

CoQ10 and Cardiovascular Disease (The Energy Times Medicine Chest) Long Beach, CA, 1995. p. 55-56.

Crayhon, R., "Energy Therapy," *Total Health*, Vol 20. No 1, St. George, Utah, Feb/March, 1998, p.14-16.

Davis, J.M., et.al., "Possible Mechanisms of Central Nervous System Fatigue Exercise", *Med. Sci. Sports Exer.* 29, 1 (1996): 45.

Depres, J.P., Bouchard, C., et.al., "Level of Physical Fitness and a Dipocyte Lipolysis in Humans," *Applied Physiology Respiratory, Environmental, and Exercise Physiology*, 56: 1157-1161, 1984.

Drake, D., Uhlman, M., *Making Medicine, Making Money*, Andrews and McMeel Publishing, 1993.

Duncan, L., *Increase Your Vitality*, Nature's Secret, Boulder, CO, 1995.

Eisenberg, D.M., et al. "Unconventional Medicine in the United States", *The New England Journal of Medicine*, 1993: 328:246-52.

Energy Times Magazine, "Energetic Explanations," Vol.9., No. 7, Long Beach CA, July/Aug., 1997, p.60.

Fernstrom, J.D., "Dietary Amino Acids and Brain Function", *Journal of The American Dietetic Association*, Vol. 94 No 1, 1:94:71-77.

Fernstrom, J.D., Wurtman, R.J., et.al., "Diurnal Variations in Plasma concentration of tryptophan, tyrosine, and other neutral amino acids: effect of dietary protein intake", *American Journal of Clinical Nutrition*, 1979; 32: 1912-1922.

Fitch, C.D., Mueller E.S., "Experimental Depletion of Creatine and phosphocreatine from skeletal Muscle", *Journal of Biol. Chem.* 1974; 149, 1060-63.

Folkers, K., et.al., *Biomedical and Clinical Aspects of Coenzyme Q (Vol.I)*, Eignevier Science Publishers, 1977.

Foster, S., and Chohgxi, Y., *Herbal Emissaries! Bringing Chinese Herbs To The West*, Healing Art Press, Rochester VT, 1992.

Foster, "Making Wise Choices in Herbal Energy Boosters", *Better Nutrition For Todays Living*, Atlanta, GA, 1995, p.66-69.

Foster, S., *Herbs For Your Health*, Interweave Press, Loveland, CO, 1996.

Global Health Publications, *The Vitamin Herb Guide*, Global Health LTD., Alberta Canada, 1987.

Greenfire, *Mainstreaming Alternative Medicine*, The Delaware Valley Directory of Alternative Health Resources, Phila Pa., Spring/Summer, 1996, No.2, p1.

Harriman, S., *The Book of Ginseng*, Jove Publishing, New York, NY, 1978.

Hobbs, C., "Overcoming Chronic Fatigue", *Veggie Life*, Concord, CA, 1:98: 56-59.

Howell, E., *Enzyme Nutrition, The Food Enzyme Concept*, Avery Publishing, Garden City NJ, 1985.

Jacob, S., et.al., "The Antioxidant-lipoic acid enhances insulin stimulated glucose metabolism in insulin-resistant rat skeletal muscle", *Diabetes*, 1996; 45: 1024-1029.

Kertzweil, P. Daily Values, "Encourage Healthy Diet", Found in *FDA Consumer*, Focus of Food Labeling, Rockville, MA, 1993, p.40-43.

King, B.C., Showers, M.J., *Human Anatomy and Physiology*, W.B. Saunders Co., Phila PA., 6th ed, 1969.

Krail, K., *Natural Stimulants, Health Food Business How*, Mark Publishing, Inc., Elizabeth, NJ, 1:91:51-52.

Lee, W.H., *Amazing Amino Acids*, Keats Publishing, New Canaan, CT, 1984.

Leibovitz, B., *Carnitine: The Vitamin Bt Phenomenon*, Dell Publishing Inc., 1984.

Lenard L., "Introducing 5-HTP Depression Anxiety and Sleep Break Through". *Life Enhancement News*, Issue 20. 10:96: 1-5.

Levy, D., "Cardiologists Take Vitamins But Don't Recommend Them", *The American Journal of Cardiology* (June 1997, Vol. 79, 1558-1500), excepted from *Alternative Medicine Digest*, Tiburon, CA., Nov. 1997, Issue 20, p.128.

References

Majeed, M., Citrin: A Revolutionary Herbal Approach to Weight Management, New Editors Publishing, Burlingham, CA, 1994.

Mindell, E., What You Should Know About Herbs For Your Health, Keats Publishing, New Cannan, CT, 1996.

Mindell, E., Earl Mindell's Herb Bible, Simon and Schuster, New York, NY, 1992.

Mindell, E., Vitamin Bible, Warner Books, New York, NY, 1991.

Morter, T.M., Your Health Your Choice, Lifetime Books, Hollywood, FL, 1995.

Murray M., Pizzorno, J., Encyclopedia of Natural Medicine, Prima Publishing, Rocklin CA, 1991

Nettle, F., and Carrol, J., How To Do Your Protein Arithmetic, Xipe Press, Carson City, NV, 1995 p.10.

Packer, L., et.al., "Alpha-Lipoic Acid as a Biological Antioxidant", Free radical Biol. Med., 1995: 19: 227-250.

Passwater, R.A., Lipoic Acid: The Metabolic Antioxidant, Keats Publishing, New Canaan , CT, 1995.

Pearson, D., Shaw, S., Life Extension, Warner Books, New York, N.Y, 1982.

Phillips, B., Sports Supplement Review, 3rd ed, Mile High Publishing, Golden CO, 1997.

Readers Digest, Magic and Medicine of Plants, Pleasantville, NY, 1986.

Redmon, G.L., Minerals: What Your Body Really Needs and Why, Avery Publishing, Garden City Park, NY, 1999.

Robertson, R.J., and Stanko, R.T., et. al., "Blood Glucose Extraction as a Mediator of Perceived Extertion During Prolonged Exercise". European Journal of Applied Physiology 61: 100-105.

Rogers, L.L., Pelton, R.B., "Glutamine in the Treatment of Alcoholism", Journal of Biological Chemistry, 1955, 214; 503-506.

Sahelian, R., Tuttle, D., Creatine: Nature's Muscle Builder, Avery Publishing Group, Garden City Park, New York, 1997.

Schofield, L., "The Art and Science of Standardized Herbal Extracts", Vitamin Retailer, East Brunswick, NJ, 4:98: 29-37.

Shook, E., Advanced Treatise In Herbology, Trinity Center Press, Beaumont CA, 1918.

Slater, A.F., Kritchevsky, D., Nutrition and The Adult Macronutrients, Plenium Press, New York, 1980.

Somer, E., "Do Your Really Need Supplements?", Shape, Woodland Hills CA, 3:98: 86-91.

Stanko, R.T., Adibi, S.A., "Inhibition of Lipid Accumulation and Enhancement of Energy Expenditure by the addition of Pyruvate and Dihydroxyacetone to a rat diet", Metabolism 35 (1996): 182-186.

Teitelbaum, J., *From Fatigued To Fantastic*, Avery Publishing, Garden City, NY, 1996.

Thorpe, K.E. "How Americans Perceive the Health Care System", National Coalition on Health Care, Washington, D.C., 1-97.

Vaugh, L., *The Complete Book of Vitamins and Minerals*, Rodale Press, Enmaus, PA, 1988.

Wade, C., Carlson, *Wade's Amino Acid Book*, Keats Publishing, New Canaan, CT, 1985.

Wade, C., *Health Tonics, Elixirs and Potions For the Look and Feel of Youth*, Parker Publishing, Co., West Nyack, NY, 1971.

Walker, N.W., *Fresh Vegetable and Fruit Juices*, Norwalk Press, Prescott, AZ, 1970.

Weil, A., *Health and Healing*, Houghton Mifflin Company, Boston, MA, 1995, p. 107-110.

Ulene, A., Ulene, V., *The Vitamin States*, Ulysses Press, Berkley, CA, 1994.

Weiner, M., *More Precious Than Gold: Enzymes*, Gero Vita Laboratories, Toronto Ontario, Canada.

Williams, S.R., *Essentials of Nutrition And Diet Therapy*, C.N. Mosby Co., St Louis, MO, 1978.

Ziglar, W., *The Ginseng Report*, International Institute of Natural Health Sciences, Inc., Huntington Beach, CA, 1979.

Chapter Six

Bailey, B.K., Jones, S.S., "Ten Ways To Increase Metabolism". *Let's Live Magazine*, Los Angeles, CA, August, 1994, p.18-22.

Berger, S., *Forever Young*. William Morrow and Co., Inc. New York, NY, 1989.

Chopra, D., *Ageless Body Timeless Mind*. Harmony Books, New York, NY, 1993.

Davis, F., *Living Alive*. Doubleday and Co., Inc. Garden City, NY, 1980.

FDA Consumer, The Magazine of the U.S. Food and Drug Administration. Rockville, MD, May 1993.

Fitzgerald, N., *Raw Glandular Supplementation: A Nutritional Approach*. Nutri-Books, Denver, CO, 1983.

Follis, R., *Deficiency Diseases*. Charles C. Thomas, Springfield, IL, 1958.

Fredericks, C., *Arthritis: Don't Learn To Live With It*. G.P. Putnam, New York, NY, 1985.

Gormley, J.J., "Chronological Age Is Irrelevant If You Maintain A Healthy Lifestyle". *Better Nutrition*, Vol. 58, No. 4, New York, NY, April 1996, p.28-30.

References

Kamen, B., "Understanding The Antioxidant Revolution: Don't Let It Start Without You". *Let's Live Magazine*, Los Angeles, CA,Oct., 1994, p.27.

Kronhausen, E., Et Al., *Formula For Life, The Antioxidant Free Radical Detoxification Program*. William Morrow, New York, NY, 1989.

Lee, W.H., *Amazing Amino Acids*. Keats Publishing, Inc., New Canaan, CT, 1984.

Mayer, J., *Human Nutrition*. Charles C. Thomas, Springfield, IL, 1964.

Mindell, E., *Live Longer and Feel Better With Vitamins and Minerals*. Keats Publishing, Inc., New Canaan, CT, 1994.

Passwater, R.A., *Selenium as Food and Medicine*. Keats Publishing, New Canaan, CT, 1980.

Pearson, D., Shaw, S., *Life Extension: A Practical Scientific Approach*. Warner Books, Inc., New York, NY, 1991.

Slobody, L.B., *The Golden Years: A 12 Step Anti-Aging Plan for a Longer, Healthier and Happier Life*. Greenwood Publishing Group, Westport, CT, 1996.

Weiner, M., *Maximum Immunity*. Houghton Mifflin, Boston MA, 1986.

Willix, R.D., *You Can Feel Good All The Time*. Health For Life, Baltimore, MD, 1994.

Chapter Seven

Atkinson, H., *Women and Fatigue*, G.P. Putnam and Sons, New York, NY, 1985.

Brown, B.B., *Supermind: The Ultimate Energy*, Harper and Row, 1980.

Earle, R., Emrie, D., and Archbold, R., *Your Vitality Quotient*, Warner Books, New York, NY, 1989.

Girdano, D.A., Everly, G.S., Dusek, D.E., *Controlling Stress and Tension: A Holistic Approach*, 3rd ed., Prentice Hall, Englewood Cliffs, NJ, 1990.

Insel, P.M., and Roth, WT., *Core Concepts In Health*, Mayfield Publishing, Co., Mountain View, CA, 1988.

Jensen, B., *The Science and Practice of Iridology*, Bernard Jensen International, Es Condido, CA, 1952.

Klatz, R., and Khalsa, D.S., "Take Two-Longevity Test", *Total Health*, Vol. 22., No. 4, Total Health Holding, St. George, Utah, Sept./Oct., 1999, p. 30-33

Maharishi, Ayur-Ved, *Fundamentals of Maharishi Ayur-Ved*, Maharishi Ayur-Ved International, Inc., Lancaster, MA, 1993, p. 1.

McQuade, W., and Aikman, A., *Stress*, E.P. Dutton and Co., New York, 1974.

Neuernberger, P., *Freedom From Stress*, Himalayan International Institute of Yoga Science and Philosophy Honesdale, PA, 1981.

Selye, H., *Stress Without Distress*, J.B. Lippincott Co., Phila, PA, 1974.

Selye, H., *The Stress of Life*, McGraw-Hill, New York, NY, 1989.

Shealy, C.N., *DHEA, The Youth and Health Hormone*, Keats Publishing, 1996.

Chapter Eight

Bandura, A., "Self-Efficacy Mechanism in Human Agency". *American Psychologist*, 1982. pp 122-147.

Berger, S.M., *Forever Young*. William Morrow and Co., Inc., New York, NY, 1989.

Chopra, D., *Boundless Energy*. Random House, Inc., New York, NY, 1995.

Dalziel, M.M., and Schoonover, S.C., *Changing Ways*. American Management Association, New York, NY, 1988.

Davidson, J.F., *Blow Your Own Horn*. The Berkley Publishing Group, New York, NY, 1987.

Farquhar, J.W., *The American Way of Life Need Not Be Hazardous to Your Health*. Addison-Wesley, Reading, MA, 1987.

Geer, J.H., Davison, G., and Gatchel, R., "Reduction of Stress in Humans Through Non Vertical Perceived Control of Aversive Stimulation". *Journal of Personality and Social Psychology*, 1970; (16): 731-738.

Girdano, D.A., Everly, G.S., Dusek, D.E., *Controlling Stress and Tension: A Holistic Approach*. Prentice Hall, Englewood Cliffs, NJ, 3rd Ed., 1990.

Matheny, K., and Cupp, P., "Desirability and Anticipation as Moderating Variables Between Life Change and Illness". *Journal of Human Stress*, 1983; (9): 14-23.

McConkey, D.D., *How To Manage By Results*. American Management Association, New York, NY, 1983.

Morris, S., "A Strong Body is a Matter of Holistics". *Health Food Business*, Melville, NY., Feb. 1989, p. 38-40.

Natelson, B.H., *Facing and Fighting Fatigue: A Practical Approach*. Yale University Press, New Haven, CT, 1998.

Padus, E., *The Complete Guide to Your Emotions and Your Health*. Rodale Press, Emmaus, PA, 1986.

Peters, T.J., and Waterman, R.H., *In Search of Excellence*. Harper and Row, New York, NY, 1982.

Podell, R.N., Doctor, *Why Am I So Tired?* Pharos Books, New York, NY, 1987.

Rosenthal, N., "Diagnosis and Treatment of Seasonal Affective Disorder". *Journal of the American Medical Association*, 270, 12:8:93: 2717-2720.

Schmidt, M.A., *Tired of Being Tired, Overcoming Chronic Fatigue and Low Energy*. Frog, LTD., Berkley, CA, 1995.

Teitelbaum, J., *From Fatigued to Fantastic*. Avery Publishing Group, Garden City Park, NY, 1996.

References

Theobold, R., *The Rapids of Change*. Knowledge Systems, Inc. Indianapolis, IN, 1987.

Ways, P., *Take Charge of Your Health: The Guide to Personal Health Competence*. The Stephen Green Press, Lexington, MA, 1985.

Index

Molecules, 31

Mood energy connection
food, 63–64, 66
and St. John's Wort, 111

N

NADA (nicotinamide adenine dinucleotide), 86
benefits of, 87
and immunity, 86–87
recommendations for, 87

National Academy of Science, 44, 48

National Cancer Institute, 52, 132, 139

National Institute of Health (NIH), 89
Office of Alternative Medicine, 80

National Institute on Aging, 132

National Research Council, 47

Natural energizers, 77–128
questions about, 80–81

Natural Sweet Raw Juice recipe, 174

Nature
invisible hand of, 130, 140
master plan of, 26
unity in, 24–25

Neiper, Dr. Hans, 153

Neurotransmitter levels, influence of nutrition on, 63

New England Journal of Medicine, 78

Niacin, 117

Nicotinamide adenine dinucleotide.
See NADA

NIH. See National Institute of Health

Nitrogen balance, 48–49

Norepinephrine levels, 63, 86, 95, 109–110

Nuclear membrane, 22

Nucleoli, 22

Nucleoplasm, 22

Nucleus, 20–22

Nuernberger, Dr. Phil, 147–148

Nutrients. *See also* Phytonutrients
accessory, 81

Nutrition
classes of, 41
influence on neurotransmitter levels, 63
proper, 39–76
recommendations for improving, 160–166
unlocking energy potential with, 56–57

Nutritional needs
guidelines for, 64
individual variation in, 49–52

Nutritional therapy, 76

O

Office of Alternative Medicine, 80

Organelles, cellular, 20–23

Organically grown food, 50

Organizations list, 189–190

Oxidative reduction, 24
activating, 31–32
catabolic, 29, 31
problems with, 138–139

Oxygen, 31

P

Packer, Dr. Lester, 82

Pantothenic acid, 117

Parkinson's disease, 87

Pauling, Dr. Linus, 62, 136, 159

Pedersen, Dr. Peter, 116

Perlmutter, Dr. David, 134

Pfeiffer, John, 17–18, 20, 23, 34

Phagocytosis, 86

Phenylalanine, 95

Phosphates, formation of, 35

Phosphorus, 119

Phosphorylation, 33

Photosynthesis, 8–9, 12

Phytonutrients, 133

Plan
  recommendations for, 160–166
  setting up, 154–156
  tracking, 166–167

Plants, as a factory, 8–9, 13

Potassium, 119

Potential energy, 5–16. *See also* Energy potential

Powerplant, internal, 34

Pro-immunity foods, 178

Proteins, 42, 48–49
  breaking down, 24
  recommendations for, 49, 52

Protoplasm, 20–21

Pyridoxine, 117

Pyruvate, 87–88
  benefits of, 88–89
  and endurance, 88
  recommendations for, 88–89

Q

Questionnaires, food-mood, 64–65

R

Radiant energy, 8–11
  electrical energy from, 11

Ratios. See Calorie ratios

Raw Juice Heart Tranquilizer recipe, 175

RDA. *See* Recommended dietary allowance

RDI. *See* Reference daily intake

Recipes, 173–175
  Anemia and Tired Blood, 175
  Casanova Cocktail, 174
  Energy Elixir, 173
  Heart-Health Revitalizer, 174
  Natural Sweet Raw Juice, 174
  Raw Juice Heart Tranquilizer, 175
  Yeast Cocktail, 174
  Young Vigor Tonic, 173

Recommendations. *See also* Food Guide Pyramid
  for alpha-lipoic acid, 83
  for antioxidants, 139–140
  for Branch Chain Amino Acids, 94
  for carbohydrates, 45
  for carnitine, 95
  for creatine, 85–86
  for fats, 46–47, 52
  for ginseng, 108–109
  for glutamine, 98
  for improving nutrition, 160–166
  for licorice, 110
  for NADA, 87
  for a plan of action, 154–157
  for proteins, 49, 52
  for pyruvate, 88–89
  for St. John's Wort, 111–112
  for sugar, 52
  for supplementation, 126–128
  for tyrosine, 96

Recommended dietary allowance (RDA), 44, 51

Reference daily intake (RDI), 44

Resistance stage of stress syndrome, 147–148

Responsibility, accepting, 158–159

Riboflavin, 117

Ribosomal RNA, 22

Ribosomes, 22

Richard, Dr. Earle, 146

RNA. *See* Ribosomal RNA

Rosenman, Ray, 144

Roth, Walton T., 143

S

St. John's Wort, 111–112
  benefits of, 111
  recommendations for, 111–112

Saltos, Elta, 50

Tyrosine, 63, 95–96
  benefits of, 96
  recommendations for, 96

U

U. S. Department of Agriculture,
    50–52, 134
  Food Safety and Inspection
    Service, 52
Ubiquinone. *See* Coenzyme Q10
UFAs. *See* Unsaturated fatty acids
Ulene, Dr. Art, 113
The Unity and Diversity of Life, 34
Unity in nature, 24–25
Universal energy molecule. *See*
    Adenosine triphosphate (ATP)
Unsaturated fatty acids (UFAs), 46

V

Vanadium, 119
Vitamin co-factors, 135–136
Vitamins, 43, 52, 113–118, 136
  A, 116
  the "ACES," 135
  B, 117–118
  E, 118
Von Liebig, 7

W

Walker, Dr. Norman W., 120, 123
Water, 43
Weaknesses, internal, 50
Web sites, 190
Weil, Dr. Andrew, 17, 142, 170
Whole food factors, 120–122
Wilkening, Virginia, 53
Williams, Dr. Sue Rodwell, 43, 90
Willix, Dr. Robert, 133, 141
Wilson, Mitchell, 3, 73
World Health Organization, 102
Wurtman, Dr. Judith, 63–64

X

Xenobiotics, 124

Y

Yeast, 121
Yeast Cocktail recipe, 174
Young Vigor Tonic recipe, 173

Z

Zinc, 119

ABOUT THE AUTHOR

Dr. Redmon was born in Edenton, North Carolina and has resided most of his life in Philadelphia, Pennsylvania. He graduated with honors and earned his Bachelors Degree in Health in 1974 from Fayettville State University. He was also honored as a member of Who's Who Among College Students in America that same year.

In addition to the above, Dr. Redmon is a graduate of the Clayton College of Natural Health (N.D.), the American Holistic College of Nutrition (Ph.D) and also received his Ph.D in Administration and Management from Walden University.

Dr. Redmon has developed a 20-year career specializing in vitamins and holistic health care within the vitamin and natural health care industry. He has served as a Regional and National Education Director for General Nutrition Centers, Inc., the largest retailer of vitamins in the United States and has had work published in numerous magazines and has been the guest speaker on several syndicated radio health programs. He is also the author of *Managing And Preventing Arthritis: The Natural Alternatives* (Hohm Press), *Minerals: What Your Body Really Needs And Why* (Avery), and *Managing And Preventing Prostate Disturbances: The Natural Alternatives*, (Hohm Press).

Dr. Redmon is a member of the Herbal Healer Academy, the Doctoral Association of New York Educators, the Holistic Health

Association of Princeton, New Jersey and the Tri-state Holistic Health Association. Additionally, he serves as an Advisory Board Member to the Clayton College of Natural Health, is an Adjunct Faculty Member (Adult Health Education) with the Washington Township Public School System in Sewell, New Jersey and serves as President of the Board of Directors for the Gallery Markey East Mall Merchants Associations in Philadelphia, PA.

Dr. Redmon currently resides in Sicklerville, New Jersey, with his wife, Brenda, and their son, George Jr.